**The Men's Hair Book: A Male's Guide To Hair Care, Hair Styles, Hair Grooming,**

**Hair Products and Rocking It All Without The Baloney**

# Table of Contents

# Preface

This book has been a long-term project of mine that I have ensured to fill up with all the answers needed for a male to get his hair looking its best.

My name is Rogelio and I'm the author of a few hair-related successful projects. I'm the founder of Manly Curls and Men's Hair Blog, 2 popular haircentric websites that cover all about hair for males as well as men's lifestyle. I'm also the author of the Amazon bestseller The Curly Hair Book: Or How Men Can Now Rock Their Waves, Coils And Kinks; a book that not only covers hair care but also provides much motivation and inspiration for those men with the toughest of manes to deal with. I myself have hard-as-rock curly hair, and I have been helping men with their hair both online and offline for a few years now.

I'm a hair nerd. Really, I am. Some people like video games, others like painting; well, I like hair. Ok, I like other stuff such as writing (this book, my book and my sites), Olympic weightlifting (have competed in a few countries), bodyboarding (love big waves) and travelling (have lived in 5 countries and traveled to many more); but, for 11 years now, I have also been on a peculiar crusade to know as much as I could about hair. This book is the result of my many experiments and experiences, both with my hair and the hair of others, so, with this book, you're not only getting the "theory" side to hair but also the "practice" side; and by that I mean that you are getting all the useful stuff that works and that I have learnt throughout the years while you are also avoiding all the useless Mickey-Mouse stuff that doesn't work and that I have had to also learn throughout the years. In other words, this book is your one ticket to having great-looking, convenient hair.

In this book, you will find that, at the end of each chapter, I relate the chapter's content to a case study; this has been thanks to my good friend and former professional barber Anthony, with whom I have had a friendship for years now and with whom I have discussed all about hair during many late evenings. While he has retired from the ancient barber profession, Anthony was keen to collaborate with me for this book, and I have related the content of every chapter to real-life cases that have occurred at Anthony's barbershop in the past so that you see how what you've learnt works in the real world.

With regards to my chosen writing style, if you already know me from my works, you will know that I write in a user-friendly, approachable and direct style; I have made it my goal to never put your testosterone levels at risk in the name of better hair, and I have written this book from the male perspective that seeks cosmetics results and convenience. Furthermore, you will find that I have written this book in British English (thus I spell -ise, not -ize) although I have aimed to keep the writing neutral so that my message gets across regardless of your English variant. Lastly, I write, instead of spell, numbers; this way you can spot them easier (e.g. 2 instead of two).

Overall, it is imperative for you to approach your hair from a systematic perspective, putting the actions that you implement for your hair into steps that will pave the path for your ultimate goal: great-looking, convenient hair that you are finally happy with. Thus, what is to follow in the next 250+ pages is a complete detailing of how to groom, care and style your hair while conveniently blending it into your modern-male lifestyle.

Let's get going.

# Acknowledgements

Having lived in 5 countries, I've met a lot of people; and I've always strived to establish and maintain relations. It's incredible how, by interacting with others, you can appreciate the true nature of the human being. After all, we humans are social creatures, and we live in a society that encourages bonding with others so as to create, inspire, motivate and yield.

I'm thankful for having bonded with so many people throughout the years, and I would not be where I am if it wasn't for the support, love and encouragement of certain people. Writing a book is a whole adventure in its own right, and it requires blood, sweat, guts and some wrist tendinitis too; thus, it is here where I'd like to thank those of you who have gifted me with your human touch in the period that it has taken me to write this book and, of course, over all these years too. You all know who you are, so thank you. Furthermore, I'd like to specifically thank the following:

- <u>You:</u> this book is for you. Every word I've written has been based on my premise of, "how does this benefit the person who has purchased my book". My goal is to deliver a literary resource (i.e. this book) that provides a solution to you; my solution is to allow you to achieve great-looking hair that can be conveniently adapted to your lifestyle as a male. What this means is that this is your book and that you are reading words that are aimed to provide you with the ability to achieve said solution; a solution that can be summarised in 3 words: "great-looking" "convenient" "hair". Thank you for placing your trust in me and for believing in my message.

- <u>A special person:</u> let's call her "cute chick". It so happens that "cute chick" has been my divine source of strength, inspiration, motivation, support, love, self-actualisation and human touch. Without "cute chick", Mr. Samson would not be Rogelio. I will always appreciate your human touch, cute chick; and no matter what in the future, I will always thank you for being, well, for being my "cute chick" and a most beautiful person. Everything about you is perfect, and I'm so thankful to have crossed paths with you in my life.

# 1) Introduction: You've Got Hair, So Do Something About It!

As modern males, we live in a society that encourages the seeking of fast results. From fat-loss pills that put your health in danger to money-making tutorials that all they do is leave you with your pockets empty, we males are every day tempted to look for shortcuts or easy ways out; and this includes our hair too.

Time and time again I've heard guys complain about their hair; what's worse is that their complaints are caused by a lack of knowledge that has them falling into a negative loop when it comes to their hair. Through TV, magazines and the Internet, we are bombarded every day with images of uber-cool hairstyles that are the result of a professional hairstylist and generous amounts of Photoshop retouching; we then brainwash ourselves into thinking that having such hairstyles is the way to go so as to be a modern, hip, trendy, metrosexual, good-looking and what-not male living in a society that pressures us into being better looking, looking younger, having more muscle and having more money; all while living the "playa" lifestyle.

Like all things in life, if you want to truly succeed in something, you need to put an effort into it and learn all there is to it. Let's think big for a second, do you think Bill Gates would have got so far had he not known so much about computers in the '80s? How about Brad Pitt, do you think he would have been so successful as an actor had he not taken acting classes early in his career and rehearsed and then rehearsed some more? Or what if Kofi Annan, a successful former Secretary-General of the United Nations, hadn't worked hard to educate himself in the '50s and become one of the most influential 20th-century diplomats despite being born in Ghana and in an era of widespread racism? Well, hair is no different (barring magnitudes, of course!), and, to have a great-looking mane atop your head, you need to study it, practise with it and put yourself to the task.

Now, knowing your hair is not that difficult. In fact, it is relatively easy provided you follow an order and a structure. Through the years, I have experimented plenty with my hair and the hair of others, and I have obtained results for myself and for others by following a system; I call this system the "hair-management equation", and it integrates 3 parts that are worked holistically to totally revamp and optimally address your hair so as to have it looking its best.

Just like Brad Pitt had to go to acting classes and rehearse plentifully to become a great actor, you will study your hair and get practising with it so as to become your hair's best expert. The key point to obtaining great-looking hair is to abide by your hair-management equation at all times, aiming to see your hair management as a system that follows an order and that has actions implemented throughout so as to give you a customised solution for your hair.

## The hair-management equation

Even if you don't realise it, you already manage your hair in one way or another. Spreading some hair gel on it, shampooing it or putting it into a hairstyle, every day you manage your hair, albeit your management is more than likely erratic and flawy; this is because the information around that we find with regards to managing our hair puts a lot of emphasis on the styling part (e.g. buying hair products and trying Mickey-Mouse hairstyles) above the rest of other parts that should otherwise make up the proper management of your hair (i.e. your hair-management equation).

This is how the Merriam-Webster dictionary describes the word "manage":

1. to handle or direct with a degree of skill: as

   a) to make and keep compliant

   b) to treat with care

The proper management of your hair entails not only skilfully handling your hair every day and looking after it (i.e. care) but it also entails keeping your hair complaint, for your hair inherently expresses itself as it wants to, not as you want it to express. So to speak, you have to dominate the beast, and, to do this, you have to know your hair to a T and approach its management in a systematic manner; all of this being what I call the "hair-management equation".

The hair-management equation is a pioneering system that I developed that sees the management of your hair as being composed of 3 equally-important aspects: hair profiling, hair grooming and hair care. Essentially, the premise to this system is that your hair is composed of 3 aspects that create synergies when integrated into each other and worked holistically (i.e. together). What's more is that these 3 aforementioned aspects are to be learnt and applied through that precise order (i.e. hair profiling, then hair grooming, then hair care), studying each aspect at a time so as to be able to move on to the next. This is what the Merriam-Webster dictionary has to say about the word "aspect":

1. a particular status or phase in which something appears or may be regarded

Indeed, your hair-management equation is composed of phases that make their appearance to holistically give you the ability to manage your hair successfully and have the best-looking hair that you can possibly own. Ergo, your hair-management equation is a mere sum of the 3 aspects: hair profiling, hair grooming and hair care, for which the total equates great-looking, convenient hair.

Visually, this is your hair-management equation:

*Hair profiling + Hair grooming + Hair Care = The best-looking hair that you can possibly own*

Figure 1 – The hair-management equation

| HAIR-MANAGEMENT EQUATION | | |
|---|---|---|
| **Hair profiling** | **Hair Grooming** | **Hair care** |
| Hair basics | Cleaning | Dry hair |
| Hair type | Conditioning | Tangled hair |
| Hair lengths | Styling | Hair loss |
| Curl Factor | Hair grooming routine | Proactive/Reactive measures |
| Norwood stage | Hair products | Nutrition |

Hair profiling refers to knowing the basics of your hair and its hows and whys (i.e. profiling) so as to then be able to understand, optimise and customise your hair grooming and hair care. The hair-profiling aspect of your hair-management equation is made up of a number of elements that make up the essence of your hair; a whole chapter (next one) is devoted to all there is about profiling your hair and you will learn how your hair is a "type", has certain "lengths", has a "Curl Factor" and is at a "Norwood" (i.e. balding) stage. Hair profiling also looks at the basics of your hair in terms of what constitutes a hair strand as well as the reason and use of the sebum secreted from your follicles, the latter being a key element in your hair-grooming aspect.

Hair grooming refers to your daily interaction with your hair so as to give it your desired state. Hair grooming, as integrated into your hair-management equation, is composed of 3 stages that are implemented every day: cleaning, conditioning and styling. These 3 stages are main actions themselves, and each stage has a set of secondary actions (i.e. actions inside the main actions) that are to be implemented. The hair-grooming aspect is customised to your own particular case based on the elements of your hair profiling, and you will build your own hair-grooming routine and schedule that will call for the 3 hair-grooming stages to be implemented every day.

Hair care refers to the strategy that you will have so as to ensure that your hair remains healthy and in the desired state that you want it to remain in over the long term. The hair-care aspect deals with, what I call, the Big 3 issues, which are 3 hair-related issues that are universally found in all males (dry hair, tangled hair and hair loss), and the hair-care aspect also deals with the nutrition needed to provide the optimal nutrients to your hair; your nutrition being the way in which to optimally look after your hair from the inside (i.e. endogenously). The addressing of the Big 3 issues via hair-care measures and via your nutrition then makes up your hair-care strategy and thus hair-care aspect.

Altogether, your goal is to optimise your hair-management equation. With this book, you will learn and apply all there is to hair profiling, hair grooming and hair care, ultimately learning to customise the hair-management equation to your own and specific case. So as to succeed in this goal, you will embark on a journey that sees the optimising of your hair-management as a series of steps and actions that tackle each aspect at a time, starting with knowing your hair's intricacies (i.e. hair profiling) and finishing with knowing how to ensure that your hair remains atop your head for the many years to come (i.e. hair care).

Be aware that, from here onwards, I will also use the term "hair-equation system" to refer to the "hair-management equation", for the hair-management equation is indeed a system. Thus, not only in this book but also in other publications, I will use the term "hair-equation system" to refer to my pioneering system: the hair-management equation. Furthermore, you yourself can also use the term "hair-equation system" when relating to others.

## Why should you want to make the most of your hair?

Hair is a highly-visible trait of yours, so any changes you make to it (be they good or bad) will have an impact on your overall looks. Thus, by optimising the management of your hair, you will get to make positive changes that will then improve your looks and image, which will then improve your self-confidence. As superficial as it may sound, women love a good head of hair on a man and people judge you by how your hair looks. You only need to look at the latest "hot guy" that women are drooling over; chances are, he will be sporting an impressive mane, and, in such a competitive society we live in, improving your physique in whatever way possible automatically puts you at an advantage.

Having said the above, I don't want you to become a hair diva or a male who obsesses about his hair and image. This book ain't about that; this book is about showing you the way to optimally manage your hair with a systematic approach and in a methodical manner so that you can then put your hair management on auto-pilot. Most guys think that having a great-looking mane involves huge amounts of time and lots of emasculation. Nonsense, I say!

My way of managing hair is one that blends, at its core, convenience with results; this is what I now want to pass on to you with this book, and it is the way that will have you becoming motivated to truly do something about your hair. In the following chapters, you will have the fire inside of you sparked so that you stop looking for excuses and start putting the thousands and thousands of words of this book into actions. Just as importantly, you will be doing all of this without having to interfere with the rest of your life or have to make any lifestyle sacrifices. As an example, the price you have paid for this book will very soon be made back as you will save money from not buying silly hair products and from actually getting to choose the right hair professional for your hair (just to name a few ways in which you'll get your money back).

# Dead rats and buzz cuts: modern-day ailments

The "dead rat" and "buzz cut" concepts are 2 concepts that I initially coined in my book <u>The Curly Hair Book: Or How Men Can Now Rock Their Waves, Coils And Kinks.</u> They are concepts that stem from the lack of hair-specific knowledge and inspiration that we modern males currently have in today's world.

The "dead rat" concept symbolises hair that looks awful because its owner doesn't know how to look after it. I first encountered this concept when I tried growing my hair over an inch in length many years ago and my mane would look awful. This is an occurrence that is shared among many males who decide to try to do something about the stuff atop their heads but fail in their quest to better hair due to a lack of optimal knowledge of their hair. This then leads a male into a cycle of neglecting his hair because, in his mind, having great-looking and convenient hair is impossible.

The "buzz cut" concept symbolises a negative attitude towards one's hair that consists of hitting the barber every X amount of weeks to get a neat, short buzz cut. Many times, a buzz cut is the consequence of a dead rat in that a male sees that trying to do something about his hair leads to nothing positive, which then makes him build a negative view, and thus attitude, around his hair. This follicular negativity is then expressed as complete neglect towards one's hair (i.e. getting a buzz cut). Other times, a buzz cut occurs because the male just can't be bothered to do something about his hair as he has been brainwashed to believe that having great-looking hair will sacrifice his time and testosterone levels. Of course, there's absolutely nothing wrong with genuinely liking a buzz cut or getting a buzz cut to enjoy the associated convenience of this hairstyle, but a buzz cut should be just another haircut/hairstyle from many others possible for you, not just the only way to have your hair in because you have been brainwashed to believe so.

This book is about changing your view on your hair and helping you get that great-looking mane that you have always envisioned yourself to have. I will refer to the terms "dead rat" and "buzz cuts" in a playful manner in the many pages ahead, for your goal is to precisely do the reverse of what these 2 concept represent.

## Conclusion

See? It isn't as difficult as we have been made to believe; so long as, during your journey, you remain clear on what constitutes your hair-management equation and continue to implement the right actions and take the right steps, you will be on your way to having great-looking, convenient hair. It really doesn't get any simpler.

The hair-management equation is made up of 3 aspects: hair profiling, hair grooming and hair care; this equation serves as a system and is the one that delivers great-looking, convenient hair for a male. You will be going through each of the hair-management aspects as you continue reading this book, and you will be learning all of the elements, actions and steps that revolve around holistically working on the 3 aspects to yield your specific customising of the hair-management equation. Altogether, you will be embarking on a journey that optimises your hair-management equation and that has an ultimate goal: to achieve great-looking, convenient hair that you are finally happy with.

As you have been able to read, I like to refer to one's "hair" as a "mane"; the reason for this is simple: a lion has a mane to visibly and visually manifest his dominant alpha trait, and you're, in fact, doing the same by means of embarking on this hair-optimising journey. Once you achieve your great-looking mane, you will be improving your looks, which will have a direct carryover on your self-confidence and will then make you a better man. Like a lion, you need to carry yourself proud and stand apart in this competitive society, and your hair just happens to sit on top of your head and thus is a visible trait of yours; making it look its best will, indeed, set you apart and improve you as a whole. That itself is worth every minute of the journey you're about to embark on.

## Anthony's barbershop case study

Taylor was a wavy-haired 20-year-old medical student who was too busy to be managing his hair every morning. He had been coming to Anthony's barbershop every 2 weeks for the last year to get a buzz cut; he'd get a #2 (guard length) all around his head. One day, Taylor confessed to Anthony that he (Taylor) was tired of getting his head buzzed and that he only did it because it was a convenient hairstyle to sport; as a medical student, his free time was marginal and Taylor believed that doing something other than a buzz cut for his hair would equate long hours in the bathroom every morning. He could not be any more wrong, and Anthony was keen to walk him on the spot through an accelerated hair-management course when Taylor showed him an interest in getting more than just a buzz cut.

Taylor learnt that time efficiency is actually indispensable to the proper management of his hair. As you will be learning throughout this book, cosmetic results need not come at the expense of convenience, and the hair-management equation actually brings a much-needed efficient order into your everyday hair handling.

Anthony did a good job in outlining the hair-management equation to Taylor; 2 months later, Taylor had left the top of his head to grow while still coming to Anthony's barbershop to trim the sides and back of his head. By this 2-month mark, Taylor's hair had totally changed and looked great, and he himself mentioned that his hair was looking "the best ever", as he put in words. Taylor was sporting a Shaggy hairstyle (a hairstyle you'll be learning later on), and he had noticed how women were eyeing him much more in the street, in class and in nightclubs; he hardly went out due to his studying schedule, which meant that, anytime he had the time to go out and socialise, he wanted to make the most of it, and thus the convenience of having great-looking looking hair that, in the beginning, he had paradoxically deemed inconvenient!

# 2) Hair-Profiling Aspect: Get To Know Your Hair!

The hair-profiling aspect of your hair-management equation is made up of several elements that you must find out. These hair-profiling elements are your hair type, hair lengths, Curl Factor and Norwood stage. Ergo, before moving on to the hair-grooming aspect, you must have these 4 elements worked out while concomitantly garnering a solid foundation of hair knowledge; all of this is what you will be learning in this chapter and what will shape your hair grooming.

<u>Figure 2 – The 4 hair-profiling elements</u>

| HAIR PROFILING | | | |
|---|---|---|---|
| Hair type | Hair lengths | Curl Factor | Norwood stage |

Perhaps the most familiar hair-profiling element, your hair type can be any of the following 4: straight, wavy, coiled or kinky. Unfortunately, these hair-typing terms are used by people recklessly and much confusion has arisen as to what each of the 4 hair types encompass. Most notorious is the use of the term "curly" to describe a certain hair type, when in reality "curly" is a term that describes any of the 3 hair types that do not grow straight: wavy, coiled and kinky. The goal is for you to put your hair into a type because your hair type, together with your specific hair lengths, will directly influence your hair grooming.

There are 2 hair lengths: extended and visible. Furthermore and so as to make your hair grooming more efficient, your extended hair length will match a specific length category: near-shaved, short, medium or long. These 4 extended hair-length categories cover different ranges of extended hair lengths, and your extended hair-length category is of the utmost importance to your hair grooming. Because your extended and visible hair lengths are continuously changing (i.e. your hair grows non-stop), you must keep an eye on your hair so as to ensure that you are still within the same extended hair-length category as time goes by. Worry not if all of this reads confusing as you will come across a detailed section in this chapter that covers all these "length" terms and you will become familiarised with all of them very soon.

Your Curl Factor goes back to my earlier mention of there being 3 "curly" hair types (i.e. wavy, coiled and kinky) and 1 non-curly hair type (i.e. straight hair). Your particular Curl Factor will influence your ability to wear certain hairstyles and will dictate how puffy your hair will look like. Technically, your Curl Factor entails the difference between your extended hair length and your visible hair length, and it is very useful to know (again, don't worry if this sounds somewhat confusing at the moment as I will cover this concept in detail later on).

Last but not least, your Norwood stage characterises the extent to which you may be balding. We males lose our hair primarily via male pattern baldness (MPB), a form of balding that is irreversible and has to do with our peculiarities of being of the male sex (i.e. men). Just about all males, if given enough lifetime, will lose their hair; only thing is that some males may go bald in their 30s or even 20s, whereas other men would lose their hair in their 90s or beyond. Thus, in order to build an awareness around this particular form of balding, the Norwood stage is included as an element of the hair-profiling aspect.

As part of your hair profiling and as part of any interaction you may have with other males who are also on their way or have already achieved their great-looking, convenient manes, I too encourage you to put your hair into an ID that consists of labelling your hair according to the 4 hair-profiling elements. That way, you can rapidly relate to other men who are going or have gone through your very same journey.

Before going through the 4 hair-profiling elements in detail, however, it is my intention to now introduce to you the basics of hair first. As it goes, you need to know the essentials of what makes your hair, so let's start this hair-profiling chapter with knowing the basics of what actually makes the stuff atop your head, for you will need to also know this to fully optimise your hair-management equation!

## What is hair?

Hair is a type of biomaterial that our bodies produce to keep us warm and protect the skin. Hair that grows in the scalp (inner area of the head that borders you face and neck) is primarily composed of a protein called keratin, and the whole length of an individual hair is called a "strand". In the scalp, a single hair strand grows from a "follicle", a tiny pocket buried inside the scalp. The part of the hair strand that you see (i.e. the part protruding from the scalp) is commonly referred to as the "shaft", and it grows in a filamentous manner. Individual hair strands are most often found grouped together in "locks": a typical hair strand in the scalp will grow in the same direction as the hair strands that are next to it, hence dozens of hair strands typically group together to grow in the same direction and make a single lock of hair.

Figure 3 – Diagram of a hair follicle including a hair shaft, sebaceous glands and associated follicular tissue

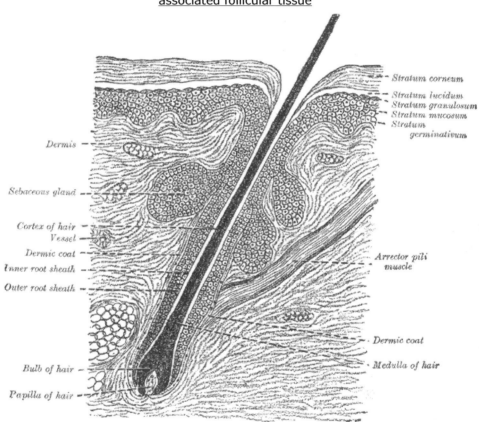

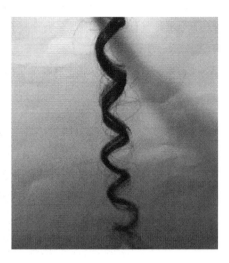

The hair shaft is composed of 3 layers: the medulla (innermost layer), the cortex (layer covering the medulla) and the cuticle (outer layer covering the medulla). The cuticle is composed of overlapping dead cells laid like shingles on a roof, and the cuticle itself is the layer of the hair shaft that we feel when we touch a given hair strand and that protects and strengthens the shaft as a whole. From now on, do note that I will use in this book the terms "strand" and "shaft" in an interchangeable manner to refer to an individual hair piece, whereas I will use the term "lock" or "hair lock" to refer to a bunch of hair strands grouped together.

The process of how a hair strand grows is that new hair material is being continuously added to the hair shaft from inside the follicle. Thus, your hair effectively grows from the follicle, and any new hair growth will be visually manifested at the base of the hair shaft (i.e. the segment closest to the scalp); hair does not grow from the tips as some people think. The good thing about the manner in which hair grows is that your hair is growing at all times to produce fresh new segments in the hair strands, so, if you cut or damage your current hair, you know that you will eventually grow new segments of the same cut or damaged strands; otherwise, we'd still be stuck with any bleaching or embarrassing hair modifications that we did to our hair in our teens!

In terms of the basics of hair, there is another essential element that you must know of, and that is scalp "sebum". The same hair follicles that hair grows from also have tiny sacks attached to them (known as sebaceous glands) that continuously secrete a natural endogenous substance resembling an oil and which is known as sebum. This oily substance is designed to coat the hair shaft, and the purpose of the sebum is to strengthen the whole hair strand and protect it from the outside elements. The end result of optimal sebum coating of the hair strands is hair that is shiny and strong, looks full and vigorous, and exudes health. Ergo, having your hair coated in your own sebum (i.e. sebuminised) is key to having great hair, but this doesn't happen on its own (especially with coiled and kinky hair), and the sebum needs to be spread manually (by you) to ensure its proper coating of your hair strands.

Hair has played an important role in our society since humans have inhabited the planet. The hair that grows from our scalp serves to protect our heads from the sun and environment, and it also serves to enhance our perceived attractiveness. Nowadays, since we have moved from caves to comfortable houses, the evolutionary role of hair has been practically lost as our exposure to the elements is much lower and beauty can be altered and faked in many ways. However, hair is still highly valued in our modern society for its beauty-enhancing properties in both women and men.

Men throughout history have worn their hair in different styles, manners and lengths, with hair coming to symbolise youth, physical vigour and prowess. From long hair to carefully-trimmed locks, men have used their hair as an indicator of their social and biological status since hair is a physical trait that is easily and instantly recognised. Centuries ago and somewhat in present day too, if you wanted to look defiant or be feared, you'd grow your hair long, and, if you wanted to be taken as a man of class, you'd wear your hair short and neat. Consequently, hair has played an important part in the social development of male status and role from past to present.

Male pattern baldness (MPB) is a type of balding almost exclusive to men, and it affects about 65% of men by age 60. MPB is a form of balding that is progressive, and it is categorised in 7 stages via the Hamilton-Norwood scale. The balding inflicted by MPB is irreversible and can hit a male at any age and of any background, although there is a strong genetic component associated to it. This is why it is so important that you do something about your hair now and learn how to manage it optimally. I always say that, sooner or later, your hair will go, so it's in your interest to make the most of it while it lasts!

Lastly, hair grows, on average, 0.5 inches (or about 1 centimetre) per month, and the rate of hair growth is affected by your diet, hormonal status and overall health. While trying to speed up your hair-growing process is quite an experimental endeavour, you can certainly and easily slow down your hair growth. Not having an optimal diet that promotes healthy hair growth, being seriously ill, or not having optimal levels of several bodily hormones can wreak havoc in the rate at which your hair grows as well as impair the quantity and quality of the hair strands.

## Hair types

There are 4 hair shapes available that a male can grow atop his head: straight, wavy, coiled and kinky. These shapes are what I term "types", and the difference between each of these 4 types is merely to do with how each type curls as it grows from the follicle, from exhibiting no curling at all (i.e. straight hair) to exhibiting very tight curling (i.e. kinky hair). What's more is that a male will grow the same type of hair all around his scalp; thus, one can successfully put his hair into a type by examining a few locks first.

It is believed that there is a "curly" gene, meaning that the expression of this gene in your DNA will influence how curly your hair will be. Hair genetics is still fairly undeveloped, and most of the scientific research surrounding hair is targeted towards hair loss, which means that, in terms of hair typing, we are left with merely being able to put our hair into a type. This curly gene is involved in giving the aforementioned range of hair-curling expressions and hence the 4 hair types available, with straight hair displaying no curling along its length to kinky hair displaying tight bends and curves along its length.

Confusion arises when using the term "curly", and some people use this term to refer to hair that is of a coiled type while others will use it to refer to kinky-growing hair. In reality, any hair that doesn't grow straight will grow curly, albeit the curling that will occur throughout the hair shaft will be of a specific grade, hence the many visual forms manifested by hair that doesn't grow straight. Essentially, curly hair can range from hair that curls slightly and forms visual wave-like shapes (i.e. wavy hair) to hair that curls tightly and forms tiny coiled shapes (i.e. kinky hair). Altogether, we thus have 2 textures of hair acting as parent groups of the hair types: non-curly (i.e.

straight hair type) and curly (i.e. wavy, coiled and kinky hair types).

<u>Figure 5 – The 2 hair textures available and their hair types</u>

| TEXTURES | |
|---|---|
| *Non-Curly* | *Curly* |
| | Wavy hair |
| Straight hair | Coiled hair |
| | Kinky hair |

Structurally, the curling (i.e. bending) that your hair may have is influenced by the cross-sectional shape of the hair shaft. In straight hair, the cross-sectional shape of the hair shaft is round whereas, in kinky hair, the cross-sectional shape of the hair shaft is almost flat. Because the structure of the hair shaft is determined genetically at the follicle level, your hair grows in the same genetically-determined shape at all times; you will always grow the same type of hair unless you go through very-specific lifetime scenarios.

Your hair type is most important with regards to your hair grooming; while all hair types share the same grooming process, the secondary actions implemented during the hair-grooming process will differ slightly according to your hair type, thus the need for you to profile your hair by means of the hair-type classification in this book. Furthermore, your ability to grow your hair longer than a medium length (i.e. 6+ inches) will be hampered somewhat depending on your hair type, with straight hair being the easiest to grow long whereas kinky hair being the most difficult to grow long.

There are several hair-typing guides available, but most guides are geared to women, not men. The only guide that is geared to men and most useful to this population is my "Curly Hair Typing Guide", which is a guide that is specific to curly hair (i.e. to the wavy, coiled and kinky hair types) and which is fully explained in my book <u>The Curly Hair Book: Or How Men Can Now Rock Their Waves, Coils and Kinks</u>. Instead, in this book, I will teach you my other hair-typing guide, which views the hair-type spectrum as composed of 4 types: straight, wavy, coiled and kinky.

To identify your hair type, all you will need to do is to inspect your hair in the mirror. A ruler may be needed, but, for the most part, you will only need your judgement as you follow the description of each type. When you find the description that most suits what you're seeing in the mirror, you will have identified your hair type.

## Why are there 4 different types of hair?

Your given hair type is due to your own genetic makeup. Your genes dictate the shape of your hair, its colour, its thickness and its rate of growth, which is why men with the same hair type will still have different-looking hair from one another. Since the hair types are based upon the shape of the hair, these are the factors that determine the shape of your hair:

- Evenness of the hair shaft: if your hair strands are built with a regular surface, your hair will be less curlier (e.g. straight hair). On the other hand, if the building blocks that make up the hair shaft are laid irregularly as opposed to evenly, your hair will bend and curve in different ranges and thus the 3 "curly" hair types, which are the wavy, coiled and kinky types.

- Cross-sectional shape of the hair shaft: the hair shaft in straight hair has a circle-like cross-sectional shape whereas kinky hair has an almost flat cross-sectional shape. The flatter the cross-sectional shape of the hair shaft is, the curlier the hair strand will be.

All in all, your hair type is dictated by your genes and you cannot change how your hair grows. However, your hair type may change permanently during critical stages of your lifetime:

- Puberty: most men find that their hair changes to a curlier hair type when they hit puberty e.g. from having straight hair during childhood to having wavy hair after having reached puberty.

- Seniorhood: there's some anecdotal evidence pointing to hair type changing in some people as they enter seniorhood although this could be mistaken for overall loss of hair density, which in some cases can make wavy hair look like straight hair, especially if the hair is kept short as with most senior males.

- <u>Exceptional distress:</u> this may cause one to not only lose his hair but also have his hair type changed.

- <u>Chemotherapy:</u> people undergoing chemotherapy to treat cancer find that they lose their hair and, when it grows back, it grows back curlier or wiry-looking.

- <u>Some medications:</u> there are a few medications used to treat severe illnesses that may alter one's hair type. It is always best that you check with your doctor.

## How to identify your hair type

Stand in front of a mirror and have your face 2 feet away from the mirror. Now, bend your head slightly forward and visualise the part of your scalp that constitutes the top of your head. From that area of your scalp, choose a lock of hair that is anywhere within the centre of your scalp. The lock of hair should be about 0.25 inches wide, and you should gently lift it up so that you can see it in the mirror.

<u>Figure 6 – Aerial view of head and area to select lock for your hair typing</u>

FRONT OF HEAD

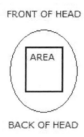

AREA

BACK OF HEAD

Once you are visualising your lock of hair, take mental notes of its shape and compare what you are able to see with the descriptions of each of the 4 hair types in the next subsection. In the case that you are unsure about your hair type from just its shape alone, get the ruler out and start measuring. If after taking measurements, you still cannot tell your hair type, then help the identifying of your hair type by using the examples of men referenced for each hair type and also work out your hair's Curl Factor, which will be explained later on in this chapter.

When visualising your hair, you should remember the ISEZ mnemonic:

- **I:** hair that is straight grows without bending, so straight-haired locks will resemble the capitalised letter I.

- **S:** hair that is wavy bends and forms waves as it grows, so wavy-haired locks will resemble the capitalised letter S.

- **E:** hair that is coiled will form spirals and coils as it grows, so coiled-haired locks will resemble the capitalised letter E (cursive form).

- **Z:** hair that is kinky will have very sharp bends and turns as it grows, so kinky-haired locks will resemble the capitalised letter Z.

The above mnemonic is very useful to keep in mind when typing your hair and also gives the hair-type guide of this book the name "ISEZ hair-type guide".

Your hair should be fully dry and without any hair products applied when attempting to identify your hair type. This specific state of your hair is best accomplished by wetting your hair in the morning (e.g. in the shower), drying your hair so that it is left damp and then going about your day until your hair reaches on its own a fully-dried state (i.e. air-dries). You should not apply any hair products to your hair once you have wetted it; your hair must be product-free in order to identify its type.

## The ISEZ hair-type guide

### Straight hair

Straight hair shows no curling (i.e. bending) whatsoever. It grows straight infinitely, hence it is very easy to spot. However, straight hair may show a slight bending at a length of over 3 inches in length, which is caused by normal wear and tear of the hair. If your hair doesn't show any signs of curling when you look at it in the mirror, your hair will be straight.

If your hair shows a very slight curling pattern (aka wave-like pattern), then get the ruler out. Ideally, use a hard ruler and, if your hair shows no curling pattern anywhere within 3 inches of length starting from the scalp, then you will be able to confirm that your hair is straight. By using a hard ruler, you will be able to simply put the lock of hair alongside the length of the ruler and check that the lock of hair follows the same straight length during the first 3 inches.

In this hair-type guide and in the rest of this book, straight hair is also referred to as Type I hair, as it resembles capitalised "i" letters as it grows. Straight hair is the hair type of Brad Pitt, Tom Cruise and Justin Bieber.

<u>Figure 7 – Representation of a straight-haired lock</u>

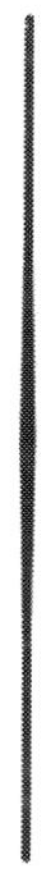

## Wavy hair

Wavy hair is hair that curls slightly, giving the visual appearance of having waves, thus the name "wavy". Wavy hair is the loosest type of curly hair (out of the 3 available), and it is hair that doesn't form coils or spirals, instead growing in S shapes and forming waves. Thus, if you spot these S shapes and wave-like shapes on your hair, you will have wavy hair.

Wavy hair that is shorter than 3 inches will be exhibiting noticeable bends and curves throughout the length of the hair strands without necessarily forming wave-like shapes. Wavy hair will not, however, form full coils or corkscrew-shapes, so, if your hair is not straight, yet no coils or corkscrew-shapes are formed, then this will indicate that your hair is of the wavy type.

Because wavy hair is a very loose curl, after all, you may have a problem telling whether you have wavy or coiled hair if your hair is very short. Thus, if your hair is shorter than 0.25 inches, it is best that you wait until your hair is a bit longer to see whether it forms waves or coils.

In this hair-type guide and in the rest of this book, wavy hair is referred to as Type S as it resembles capitalised "s" letters as it grows. Wavy hair is the hair type of George Clooney, Antonio Banderas and Adrian Grenier.

Figure 8 – Representation of a wavy-haired lock

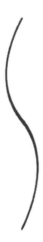

**Coiled hair**

Coiled hair is hair that curls in the shape of coils and spirals. This is the hair type that is most commonly referred to as "curly" hair, despite the fact that wavy hair and kinky hair also curl. Coiled hair is easy to spot as you will be able to see coils and spirals forming in your hair, which, with enough length, will look like cursive Es.

Figure 9 – Cursive-like capitalised "e" illustrating how coiled hair grows

Coiled hair can take up to 1 inch to form coils and spirals, and, as with wavy hair, it is best that you wait until your hair is over 0.25 inches in length to determine whether it is wavy or coiled.

In this hair-type guide and in the rest of this book, coiled hair is referred to as Type E as it resembles cursive, capitalised "e" letters as it grows. Coiled hair is the hair type of Justin Timberlake, Kenny G (the musician) and Corbin Bleu.

Figure 10 – Representation of a coiled lock

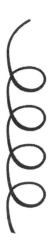

**Kinky hair**

Kinky hair is hair that curls so tightly that its coils are very hard to see, factually forming kinks (Z shapes) and coils that have very-deep bends. The main difference between coiled and kinky hair is that kinky hair does not have naturally-defined coils, and, if you have kinky hair, you will not be able to discern any hair locks making up your mane and you will find it very difficult to notice your hair's coils in the mirror without getting closer. Your hair will look like one whole unit rather than being composed of visible locks.

Kinky hair forms coils at incredibly-short lengths, thus its coils are not visible at the stipulated distance from the mirror (2 feet) that you should be away from when identifying your hair type. Typically, kinky hair will form coils and kinks within a length of 0.125 inches, which gives rise to the distinct look of kinky hair. Kinky hair is most-commonly associated with people of African heritage (e.g. Afro Americans), and it is also called afro-textured hair. Do bear in mind that kinky hair is not only limited to those men of African heritage nor is kinky hair the only hair type that an African-descending male can grow.

In this hair-type guide and in the rest of this book, kinky hair is referred to as Type Z hair as it resembles capitalised "z" letters as it grows. Kinky hair is the hair type of Lenny Kravitz, Will Smith and Kofi Annan.

<u>Figure 11 – Representation of a kinky-haired lock</u>

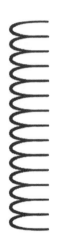

Figure 12 – Summary of the 4 hair types in the ISEZ hair-type guide

| | HAIR TYPES | | | |
|---|---|---|---|---|
| | STRAIGHT | WAVY | COILED | KINKY |
| Hair shape | Straight linear shape | Wave-like shape | Coiled and spiral-like shape | Coiled and tightly-angled shape |
| Alphabetical resemblance | I | S | E | Z |

## Hair lengths

There are 2 hair lengths available: extended length and visible length. Both hair lengths are essential to your hair-management efforts, and you should know them both. To find both of them out, you will only need either a measuring tape or a ruler; preferably a measuring tape for measuring your extended length and a hard ruler for measuring your visible length.

Because extended hair length is the most important out of the 2 lengths for your hair-grooming aspect, you will not only work out your specific extended length but you will also put your extended length into a category. Putting your extended length into a category is like putting your hair shape into a type: both hair type and extended length category are profiling elements that will be essential to determine your specific hair-grooming efforts.

Figure 13 – Makeup of the hair-lengths element

| HAIR LENGTHS ELEMENT | | |
|---|---|---|
| Extended hair length | Visible hair length | Extended length category |

## The 2 types of hair length

**Extended length**

Extended length is the length of your hair when it is in a fully-flattened state. To find out your extended hair length, choose a lock of hair from the same area of your scalp as you chose for your hair-typing efforts. Gently pull the lock of hair until any curves and bends it may have are fully flattened, and then measure the length of your hair starting from the base of the lock (i.e. scalp) right to the tip. Repeat the measuring process on 2 more locks that are next to the lock you've chosen. Then, simply work out the mean average of the 3 length results you've obtained from the 3 measured locks so as to find out your particular extended length.

Your extended hair length is the most important of the 2 length types as it will be crucial for your daily hair grooming. The 0.5 inches of hair growth that we men get every month is of extended length.

**Visible length**

Visible length is the length of your hair when it is in its natural non-flattened state. To find out your visible hair length, do as for finding out your extended length, only that, this time, you will not be flattening your hair. Gently hold the lock of hair to be measured without pulling it, for you want to find out its length as it normally has while resting on your head. Make sure that you measure a straight line from the base of the lock (i.e. scalp) to its tip, hence a hard rule will be more convenient in this case.

Visible length will differ from your extended length unless you have straight hair. Visible length is most useful for determining how long it will take you to achieve certain hairstyles denoted by a body part (e.g. shoulder length), and this particular hair length should be measured when your hair has been fully dried and hasn't had any hair products applied prior to its measuring.

## Extended length category

As has been said, the extended length of your hair is the most important as it is highly relevant for your daily hair grooming. Essentially, your hair-grooming efforts will differ somewhat according to your extended hair length as well as your hair type. However, the efforts involved in your daily hair grooming will be similar within several ranges of extended lengths, thus it is more convenient to put your extended length into a category. This way, you only need to remember the category of your hair when you are studying and optimising the hair-grooming aspect and any time that you are tweaking your hair-management equation.

There are 4 extended hair-length categories: near-shaved, short, medium and long. You should know at all times what your extended length category is, as jumping from one category to the other will mean a change in the grooming of your hair.

These are the categories of extended hair length:

## Near-shaved

This extended length category ranges from freshly shaved to 0.125 inches of extended length (or a #1 in a hair clipper). This category is the most convenient of all as it requires the least grooming.

## Short

This extended length category ranges from 0.125 inches to 2 inches of extended length. It is a category that is chosen by most males as it allows for the implementing of some creative hairstyles on one's hair, and its daily grooming is not as intensive as the longer length categories.

## Medium

This extended length category ranges from 2 inches to 6 inches of extended length. Straight hair and wavy hair will start to hang down at the extended lengths that encompass this category, whereas coiled and kinky hair will still defy gravity.

## Long

This extended length category goes from 6 inches of extended length and beyond. This category is the one that requires the most grooming efforts regardless of hair type, and, the longer the hair, the more careful one has to be with his grooming.

Coiled and kinky hair will start hanging down at 10+ inches of extended length.

Figure 14 – The 4 extended length categories

| EXTENDED HAIR LENGTH | |
|---|---|
| Hair length (inches) | Hair length category |
| Less than 0.125 | Near-shaved |
| 0.125 – 2 | Short |
| 2 – 6 | Medium |
| Over 6 | Long |

## Knowing your hair lengths

Out of the 3 hair-length elements that we have seen in this section (extended length, visible length and extended length category), the one that you should know at all times is your extended length category. Any time that you cut your hair, measure your extended hair length so as to know what your new extended length category is. Likewise, strive to measure your extended hair length every month if you haven't cut your hair in that period; this way, you can ensure that you are still remaining in the same extended length category considering that your hair will naturally grow about 0.5 inches of extended length in that month.

From now onwards, do note that any mentions of "hair length" or "length" as a generic term will be referring to extended length, not visible length. If I want to refer to visible length, I will use its full term (i.e. include the word "visible" before "length").

# Curl Factor

The Curl Factor is an interesting element of your hair that measures how strongly your hair curls, and it is essentially the difference between your extended hair length and your visible hair length expressed as a number. The Curl Factor is most relevant for the hair types within the curly texture (wavy, coiled and kinky) as the difference between extended hair length and visible hair length in straight hair is negligible.

The Curl Factor affects the ability of hair to hang down as hair that curls the most will puff out and will continue to defy gravity until it hits very long lengths. Likewise, the Curl Factor is a reliable element to know how different the look of your hair will be between its wet or damp state and its dried state (i.e. the Damp vs. Dry effect). Finally, as said in the hair-typing section, you can always use the Curl Factor to help you with your hair-typing efforts so as to precisely identify your specific hair type.

To work out your Curl Factor, divide your extended hair length by your visible hair length, with the result being your particular Curl Factor:

*Extended hair length / Visible hair length = Curl Factor*

The higher the number that you work out, the higher your Curl Factor will be, and the more it will mean that your hair curls. Straight hair will have the lowest Curl Factor (i.e. 1-1.1) while kinky hair will have the highest Curl Factor, sometimes being as high as 4 with this hair type.

Since many times the lengths of hair to be measured are very short, it is best to measure your hair via the metric system in either centimetres or millimetres; this is because a difference of a few millimetres can throw out the result you obtain for your Curl Factor. However, if you still prefer to use the imperial system (i.e. inches) to measure your hair lengths so as to work out your Curl Factor, then, by all means, do so, but bear in mind that you need precise measurements.

The following are the typical Curl Factor ranges of each of the hair types:

- **Straight hair:** 1-1.1

- **Wavy hair:** 1.11-1.5

- **Coiled hair:** 1.51-2.5

- **Kinky hair:** Over 2.51

Figure 15 – Curl Factor ranges for each hair type

| Hair type | Curl Factor |
|-----------|-------------|
| Straight hair | 1-1.1 |
| Wavy hair | 1.11-1.5 |
| Coiled hair | 1.51-2.5 |
| Kinky hair | 2.51+ |

The Curl Factor can also be used when you are unsure about your hair type. If you haven't been able to nail down your hair type through the information on the hair-type guide and you have doubts between 2 hair types, you can then use your Curl Factor to further determine your correct hair type although the Curl Factor is not foolproof and you are best combining it with the references of men used for the hair types to further identify your hair type.

The Damp vs. Dry effect is an interesting occurrence that, as aforementioned, is related to the Curl Factor. You will have noticed throughout these years of living with your hair that your mane looks different when it is damp as opposed to when it is fully dried. While not essentially related to the hair-profiling aspect of your hair-management equation, it is in your interest to put a name to this occurrence, hence the Damp vs. Dry effect.

As a rule of thumb, the higher your Curl Factor, the higher the difference in the looks of your hair between its damp and fully-dried state (i.e. more noticeable Damp vs. Dry effect). This occurrence is a natural one in that your hair is weighted down and thus elongated when your hair is damp due to the weight of the retained water and moisture in the hair strands. What this means is that your hair will be elongated and not in its natural state and visible length when it is damp. As the hair dries, either by you purposely drying your hair or as the hair air-dries alone, the hair will lose the added water weight that it gained from having wetted/dampened it and will then curl back to whatever shape it has when it is in its natural state. Thus, the higher your Curl Factor is, the more noticeable the difference between the damp state of your hair and the dry state of your hair and thus the more noticeable the Damp vs. Dry effect will be. Lastly, the longer your hair is, the more noticeable the Damp vs. Dry effect will tend to be.

Figure 16 – Damp vs. Dry effect according to hair type and extended hair length (general guideline)

| Hair length | HAIR TYPES | | | |
|---|---|---|---|---|
| | Straight | Wavy | Coiled | Kinky |
| Short | Barely | Barely | Mild | Moderate |
| Medium | Barely | Mild | Moderate | Intense |
| Long | Barely | Mild | Moderate | Intense |

The above table gives you an estimate of how your Damp vs. Dry effect will be according to your hair type and extended hair length. Your Damp vs. Dry effect can, however, differ according to what type of hairstyling product you use and how much you use of the chosen product. The hairstyling products that decrease the Damp vs. Dry effect (i.e. your dried hair will resemble your damp hair more) are styling creams, natural oils, leave-in conditioners, hair spray and strong-hold hair gel. The range of hairstyling products available to you are covered in the next chapter (hair-grooming chapter) since hairstyling products are part of your styling stage in the hair-grooming process.

Going back to the Curl Factor, your Curl Factor relates to your hair grooming because, by knowing your specific Curl Factor, you can predict how different a new hairstyle will look when you try it on and you will thus be prepared for any aesthetic changes of your hair as it fully dries.

## The Norwood stage

Every male will sooner or later start to bald. Primarily, men bald via a hair loss condition known as male pattern baldness (MPB). This type of hair loss is characterised by progressive receding of the frontal hairline (hairline bordering the forehead) with concomitant loss of hair density all over the scalp (i.e. number of hair strands per centimetre square). The receding of the frontal hairline progresses (towards the back of the head) until no hair is left on the top of the head, and this balding progression is classified in 7 advancing stages by the Norwood scale.

I will cover MPB in more detail as well as all about treating it in Chapter 4 "Hair-Care Aspect: The Big 3 Issues To Battle To Sport Great-Looking Hair". However, for now, you must identify (approximately) from the classification below what Norwood stage you're currently in. Stage I is a teenager-type hairline with no receding occurring; from there onwards, each incremental stage has further hairline recession and loss of hair density on the top of the head. To better identify your Norwood stage, compare your current hairline with the one you had when you were 12-16 years old; use 2-3 old pictures of you with the head visible so that you can get an idea of how your hairline looked at such a young age.

These are the stages visualised:

Figure 17 – The Norwood classification model with the 7 stages

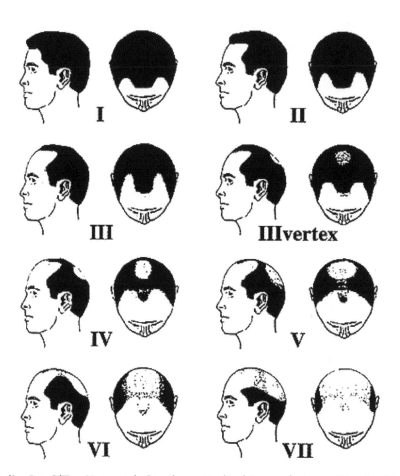

*Image credit: Dr. O'Tar Norwood, Southern Medical Journal, Issue 11, Vo. 68, 1975*

Male pattern baldness is progressive and actually starts between Stages II and III; by that point, your scalp will continue to dramatically lose more and more hair in a predictable pattern until no hair strands are left on top of the head. These are the stages themselves:

- Stage I: this is a "juvenile hairline" and is the hairline that you would have had in your early/mid teens. The frontal hairline (i.e. hairline bordering the face) is oval shaped, and the temples sit at brow level when seen from the side. Some men keep this hairline beyond their teen years while most men move on to Stage II in their late teens and early 20s.

- Stage II: this is regarded as an adult or "mature" hairline. The temples have receded slightly (about an inch) from the juvenile hairline in Stage I, yet the temples are way in front of the ears when seen from the side profile. No hair loss occurs anywhere else in the scalp and this stage does not represent balding.

- Stage III: the temples have continued to recede from Stage II and are now at ear-lobe level (when seen from the side). Likewise, the frontal top of the head has lost hair density and has too receded somewhat. This stage represents the commencement of true male pattern baldness and is the earliest Norwood stage to diagnose MPB.

- Stage III Vertex: the same frontal-hairline receding occurs as per Stage III only that, in this variant (Stage III Vertex), the vertex (crown or rear top of head) has started to bald too, leaving a bald patch in this scalp region.

- Stage IV: the receding of the frontal hairline (including temples) continues further (almost past ear level from the side), and the balding in the vertex expands circumferentially from the previous stage. There is, however, still a band of hair on the top that connects both sides of the head (acting as a "follicular bridge").

- Stage V: the receding of the frontal hairline is aggravated further and the balding in the vertex region continues to expand, to the point that the frontal receding has almost reached the balding in the vertex. The bridge of hair that was relatively free of balding in Stage IV has, by this fifth stage, started to break (i.e. further loss of hair in this remaining top segment of the scalp).

- Stage VI: there is no longer a bridge of hair connecting the sides of the head; the top of the head is now bald except for a few individual random hairs. The sides and back of the head, however, remain with the same hair density as in Stage II.

- Stage VII: in this final stage and once all the hair on the top of the head is gone, the sides and back of the head start to now bald profusely until all there is left is a narrow band of hair bordering the hairline of the ears and neck.

Guiding yourself with the diagram in Figure 17 of the Norwood classification and using the detailing of each of the Norwood stages, you should now identify which is your current Norwood stage, for your particular stage will serve to customise your hair care and range of hairstyles available to you. To carry out the identifying of your current Norwood stage, take pictures of the front, side and top of your head, and then compare those pictures to the pictures of you when you were going through puberty (12-16 years old). Try to notice any differences in your hairline and overall density, and then put yourself into a Norwood stage. I recommend you to use Roman numerals (I-VII) instead of Arabic numerals (1-7) for your Norwood stage although you may find either of these 2 numeral types used in other hair-loss literature.

Male pattern baldness has a predictable progression, though it must be said that it not always follows the pattern of hairline recession depicted in the Norwood classification model, and MPB may rarely manifest itself with generalised hair loss and little hairline recession. However, the Norwood stage classification is a fairly reliable male-baldness model (used by hair-loss specialists) and one that I urge you to put to use by identifying your Norwood stage so as to further know your hair and be able to get the most out of it and the advice in this book.

We men produce a hormone called dihydrotestosterone (DHT), which has a pro-balding effect at the hair-follicle level, essentially choking the hair follicles and causing them to permanently stop producing hair material (i.e. grow more hair). However, the impact of DHT on the follicles is determined genetically, meaning that your own genes dictate when you will start balding and how fast it will occur. About 60% of men have gone bald by age 65, and male pattern baldness can occur at any age and regardless of race or lifestyle. Likewise, the constant natural impact of DHT on your hair follicles means that, if given enough lifetime, you will start to bald. It is true that a minority of men die in their late age (e.g. in their 80s) with still a fully-visible mane, but, were they to have lived longer (e.g. 20-30 years more), their hair line would have continued to recede and more hair follicles would have ceased to produce hair (i.e. balding). It really is about winning the genetic lottery (plus some environmental factors) when it comes to being drastically affected by MPB.

Male pattern baldness should not be confused with other forms of hair loss caused by medications, stress, disease or trichotillomania (i.e. removing your hair due to anxiety or a mental disorder). Male pattern baldness is quite unique in that it is caused by DHT and your scalp's genetic disposition to DHT's long-term effects.

Male pattern baldness is the reason for my emphasis on telling guys (including you!) to wake up, smell the coffee and start addressing their hair optimally. Your hair will sooner or later go, so you might as well do something about it and maximise its years left.

## Conclusion

By now, you have all the profiling information about your hair that is needed to make the most of its grooming and caring. Let's go over what you must extract from this hair-profiling chapter:

- Know what a hair strand, hair shaft and hair lock are.

- Know that your hair follicles secrete an oily substance (i.e. sebum) that is imperative for having the best-looking hair.

- Know your hair type.

- Know your extended length, visible length and extended length category.

- Know your Curl Factor.

- Know your current Norwood stage.

Figure 18 – Depiction of the 2 textures, 4 hair types and Curl Factor

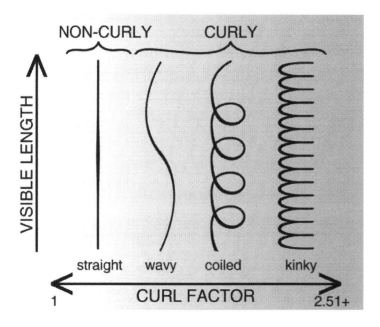

By profiling your hair, you can begin to understand that, to have great-looking hair, you must first know the stuff growing atop your head. Furthermore, from my experience, knowing the hows and whys of whatever you aim to improve is the best way to make the most of your efforts. Your hair grooming will involve your day-to-day management of your hair while your hair care will involve your long-term strategy to keep your already-achieved great mane. Ergo, you must first profile your hair so as to continue to optimise your hair-management equation with your hair-grooming and hair-care aspects. Ultimately, these 3 hair-management aspects (i.e. hair profiling, hair grooming and hair care) and their integrating are crucial to achieving your goal of having great-looking hair that will stay there for the rest of your hair strands' days (however long that may be!).

Last of all, from now on, group your particular hair-profiling elements so as to have your "hair ID". In the near future, you may want to relate to other fellow men with regards to the discussion of hair or hair-related issues, thus having a particular hair ID helps you to rapidly identify yourself and identify others. Your hair ID is made up of your:

- <u>Hair type:</u> expressed as the alphabetical letter that it is represented by in the ISEZ hair-typing guide.

- <u>Hair-length category:</u> expressed as the first capitalised letter of your specific category. Use "S" for short, "M" for medium, "L" for long. Near-shaved is expressed with the first letter of each word, so it reads as "NS" ("N"ear-"S"haved).

- <u>Curl Factor:</u> expressed as your worked-out number.

- <u>Norwood stage:</u> expressed as any of the 7 stages written in Roman numerals.

The order of the elements making up your hair ID is as listed above too, and each element is separated by a slash ("/"). For example, your hair ID could be "S/L/1.4/III" if you had wavy hair that was at a long-length category, that had a Curl Factor of 1.4 and that was at a stage III of the Norwood classification. You could also be a "Z/M/3/II" if you had kinky hair that was at a medium-length category, that had a Curl Factor of 3 and that was at a stage II of the Norwood classification. Work out your hair ID and keep it in the back of your mind for the future.

## Anthony's barbershop case study

Alexander was a 32-year old professional who liked to look sharp at all times. He came to Anthony's barbershop looking to grow his hair a bit more as he was tired of the same Crew Cut hairstyle that his other hairdresser would perform for $50. Alexander's hair was about 1 inch in (extended) length, and he had asked Anthony to tell him whether he had curly, wavy or what-it-was hair. Alexander's wife said he had wavy hair, yet he had been told repeatedly by acquaintances in the past that he had curly hair; his hairdresser told him he had "thick hair" and would leave it at that. Thus, Alexander wasn't sure of the differences in hair-typing terms that people would loosely use to describe his hair. He didn't know what to make of this whole story, and, every time he read an article of a hairstyle in a magazine, he wasn't sure if the hairstyle would suit him as the article would use hair-typing words in the same loose manner as his acquaintances would use. Overall, he was very confused about his hair, which obviously had a negative effect on his hair-management efforts.

Alexander's hair showed a noticeable bend at the 1-inch length he had. Anthony had asked Alexander if he had grown his hair in the past and if he remembered whether his hair formed coils and spirals or whether his hair formed waves. Alexander recalled having wave-like patterned hair, but he really could not give Anthony a concise answer. His hair hadn't coiled by the 1-inch length mark, so it was quite apparent that his hair was wavy, not coiled. However, because no full wavy shapes had formed yet in Alexander's hair, Anthony decided to take the ruler out and work out his specific Curl Factor to ascertain that Alexander did indeed have wavy hair.

Alexander's hair had an extended length of 28 millimetres (1.12 inches) and a visible length of 20 millimetres (0.8 inches), hence his Curl Factor was 1.4. Anthony measured in millimetres because, at such short hair lengths, it is better to use the metric system to benefit from measuring in millimetres.

Anthony was able to confirm to Alexander that he did indeed have wavy hair, and Anthony proceeded to explain to him how wavy hair is included in the spectrum of curly hair. While both Anthony and I (yours truly) are aware that many magazines use hair-typing terms loosely and without really knowing what they are, Anthony had Alexander understand why his hair was wavy through the ISEZ hair-typing guide and explained to him the rationale and method to hair profiling that you have learnt in this chapter. Alexander left extremely satisfied as he finally knew his hair, and, the next time he came back to Anthony's barbershop, he brought along a picture of Adrian Grenier sporting a hairstyle that he (Alexander) wanted to emulate. "No problem, my friend", said Anthony as he knew, by then, Alexander's hair.

# 3) Hair-Grooming Aspect: Your Daily Interacting With Your Mane

Hair grooming is the second hair aspect of your hair-management equation. It is so crucial that, without it, it doesn't matter how much you care after your hair or how much effort you've put into your hair profiling, your mane just won't get anywhere near the goal of great-looking hair.

Hair grooming revolves around your day-to-day interaction with your hair so as to clean it, condition it and style it. Normally done during your showering time, your hair grooming is a daily process that has the 3 actions of cleaning, conditioning and styling implemented as stages. Thus, your hair grooming is composed of 3 sequential stages: cleaning, conditioning and styling.

This is how you would typically groom your hair in any given day:

1. Get in the shower.

2. Soak your hair in water.

3. Use shampoo, then rinse it (first stage, cleaning).

4. Apply conditioner to your hair for 2 minutes, then rinse it (second stage, conditioning).

5. Get out of the shower.

6. Dry your hair, grab some hairstyling product and give yourself a hairstyle (third stage, styling).

7. Done!

Can you see the method and flow? As illustrated in the above 7 points, the 3 stages of cleaning, conditioning and styling are performed sequentially; that is, the stages follow from one another and are implemented in one go. Therefore, it is during your showering time that grooming your hair is best performed.

Each stage of your hair-grooming process has secondary actions; you will be selecting different secondary actions at each of the stages depending on the day that it is according to your hair-grooming schedule. To implement the cleaning stage, you can either use a shampoo or use your fingers (i.e. Sebum Coating method). To implement the conditioning stage, you can either use a conditioner, skip the conditioner and/or use your fingers to spread your own sebum. To implement the styling stage, you will dry your hair, use a leave-in conditioner, choose a hairstyling product and/or put your hair into a hairstyle.

This is how the different secondary actions pan out in each of the 3 hair-grooming stages:

Figure 19 – The 3 hair-grooming stages and their secondary actions

| STAGES | SECONDARY ACTIONS | | | |
|---|---|---|---|---|
| Cleaning | Use Shampoo | Sebum Coating method | | |
| Conditioning | Use normal conditioner | Sebum Coating method | Skip conditioning | |
| Styling | Use leave-in conditioner | Use hairstyling agent/s | Put hair into hairstyle | Dry hair |

Your goal is to dominate the 3 stages stages fully so as to be able to perform them efficiently every day. Furthermore and as has been said, each day will vary in terms of what secondary actions are implemented, yet the order and inclusion of the 3 hair-grooming stages is always abode by; every day, you will clean, condition and style your hair, albeit in different manners as per the selected secondary actions.

Your hair grooming is dependent upon your shampooing frequency. As you will learn in this chapter, you have to find out your optimal shampooing frequency, which means that, for the optimal grooming of your hair, you will use shampoo on some days (i.e. shampooing days) and you will clean your hair with your fingers on the rest of the days that you do not use shampoo (i.e. non-shampooing days). Once you have found out your shampooing frequency, you will then establish what secondary actions to

46

implement on your shampooing days and non-shampooing days, effectively building up your shampooing routine and schedule.

Most men have absolutely no clue about how to groom their hair and don't know how to properly use the different hair products available, which is why 9 out of 10 folks in any given town walk around with subpar hair. Of course, you can hit the barber or hairdresser plentifully to make up for your lack of knowledge of your hair, but, then, how useful would that be to modern males like you and I who want great-looking hair that is also convenient? If you want to own the best hair that you can possibly have, you must know and manage your hair grooming; full stop. And, unlike with women, hair grooming for males can be performed conveniently and hassle-free; this is indeed what you are going to be learning in this chapter!

## First Stage – Cleaning

Cleaning your hair is the first stage of your hair-grooming routine. When it comes to cleaning one's hair, most people think of using a shampoo. Indeed, shampoos are the best-known tools to clean your hair, but there is another form of cleaning your hair that you will be using on some days to substitute the shampoo; I have coined this the Sebum Coating method, and it involves the use of your fingers to clean the hair via the running of your fingers along the hair locks to create mechanical friction.

The problem with shampooing is that shampoos are very powerful hair-cleaning agents and using them daily is counterproductive because shampoos remove the much-needed sebum from the hair strands, which ultimately creates an instant dead rat if the shampoo is used too frequently or too much. The trick lies in scheduling shampooing days every so often and then using the Sebum Coating method to clean the hair on those days that no shampoo is used; this shampooing trick is what I call the No Shampoo method and its foundation is based upon you finding your optimal shampooing frequency and using the Sebum Coating method on your non-shampooing days. What's more is that the Sebum Coating method not only cleans the hair but also helps to spread the secreted sebum (from the follicles) along the hair strands, thus the Sebum Coating method has a strong conditioning action too.

Your hair-grooming routine will be built around your worked-out shampooing frequency. Because shampoos are so powerful, you will need to use a hair conditioner following the rinsing of the shampoo to restore the gloss of your hair. On those days that you don't shampoo (i.e. non-shampooing days), you will have the option of skipping the hair conditioner for your second stage and instead satisfy your second stage with the Sebum Coating method due to this method's dual cleaning and conditioning actions.

In summary, you will start your hair-grooming routine every day by either shampooing your hair or doing the Sebum Coating method, and, once you have finished implementing either of these 2 secondary actions for your cleaning stage, you will move on to the second conditioning stage. Altogether, the shampooing on specific days and the use of the Sebum Coating method on non-shampooing days is what I refer to as the No Shampoo method; having said that, worry not about the actual name (i.e. No Shampoo method) for this is a name I have coined so that in the future you can relate to others via the use of specific terms. From here onwards, simply focus on learning about shampooing and the Sebum Coating method.

## Shampooing

**The optimal shampooing method**

Shampoos are great hair-cleaning products. The majority of shampoos contain sulphate-type ingredients that are very efficient in removing accumulated sebum, residue from hair products and dirt from your scalp. However, shampoos will also remove the optimally-spread sebum from your sebuminised hair strands if you don't use this hair-cleaning agent properly, which is why you must know how to optimally use shampoo on your hair.

Shampoos produce lather, for which men (and women) have been brainwashed to believe that a head covered in shampoo lather equates the right way to clean one's hair. While lather is not bad per se, lather should only be left to act on the scalp and the segment of the hair strands closest to the scalp; not all over the hair, as shampoo commercials have shown us for decades. Excesses of sebum and residue from hair products are most difficult to remove from the segment of the hair strands that is closest to the scalp (i.e. the base of the shaft) and from the scalp itself, thus you must ensure that the shampoo and any lather created is left on the scalp and base of the hair strands while not coating the rest of the hair. Any dirt or residue that is on the rest of your hair is easily removed on your non-shampooing days with your fingers (i.e. the Sebum Coating method) and with running water, thus the emphasis of having the shampoo act primarily on the scalp and base of the hair shaft.

To efficiently and optimally shampoo your hair, you must do the shampooing process in a methodical manner, using your fingers to spread the shampoo on your scalp and visualising your scalp in the following 6 segments:

1. Front of the top of the head

2. Centre of the top of the head

3. Back of the top of the head (i.e. vertex)

4. Left and right sides of the head above the ears (i.e. each side is 1 independent segment)

5. Nape/lower back of the head (4 inches above the hairline of your neck)

This scalp segmenting is ideal for any time in which you need to do anything to your hair and you need to denote certain parts of the scalp. With regards to your hair grooming, this particular scalp segmentation (i.e. the 6 segments) is especially useful for your shampooing process, Sebum Coating method and for any hairstyles you choose to give yourself.

Once you are aware of the 6 segments that you can divide your scalp in, go through these chronological steps to shampoo your hair optimally:

1. Soak your hair with water.

2. Once soaked, grab the shampoo bottle and squeeze out a fingertip of shampoo.

3. Place the squeezed-out fingertip of shampoo on the centre of the top of your head.

4. Repeat Step 2 and 3 so as to place the shampoo on the remaining 5 segments of your scalp. Follow this order: front of the top of your head, vertex, each side and nape.

5. Once you complete Step 4, use the tips of your index, middle and ring fingers (joined as if making a pad) to gently massage each segment of the scalp where the shampoo rests, aiming to spread the shampoo evenly in a 4-inch radius. Do this:

   a. Work on 2 segments at a time, using each hand for each segment (remember to use the 3 fingertips making a pad).

   b. Pair the segments so as to massage them simultaneously as follows: forehead & vertex, centre of top of head & nape, and the 2 sides of the head; start in that order too.

   c. Spend 20 seconds on the paired segments and massage in a circular motion. Do not use running water as you massage; when shampooing, running water is only used to either soak your hair or to rinse the shampoo.

6. Allow the lather created in Step 5 to sit naturally on the scalp. Do not spread it any further than what has been created by the massaging motion. It is fine if some lather unintentionally covers parts of your hair locks that aren't the scalp or base of the strands, just don't actively promote the coating of your mane with lather. You want the lather to be sitting primarily on the scalp; that is, on the surface of your head's skin.

7. Once you have finished massaging the last paired segments (i.e. sides of head), use running water from the shower bulb to rinse the shampoo. Tilt your head forward or backward so that the lather is washed away effectively and without getting in your eyes.

That is it. Even when pressed for time, this shampooing method will fit in nicely in anyone's busy schedule as the most that it will take is 5 minutes, and that's being uber conservative with the time. As you learn to master the above method, you will progressively cut down the time that it takes you to implement your shampooing.

The massaging of your scalp with the shampoo will take you just 1 minute since you will be massaging 2 segments at a time for a count of 20 seconds, the complete soaking of your hair will take you 30 seconds, the messing around with placing the shampoo on your scalp will take you another 60 seconds, and the rinsing of the shampoo will take you 30 seconds (if at all). You can realistically cut down the whole shampooing process to 3 minutes once you get good at it, and you will get good at it in a short timespan once you get practising.

The main thing to remember is that you want the shampoo to do most of its work on the scalp, not along the full length of the hair strands. Secreted sebum tends to accumulate excessively on the scalp and on the base of the hair shaft, leaving the rest of the hair shaft, from mid-length to the tip, with little sebum coating, and thus the cause for dryness and brittleness commonly found in improperly-groomed hair. You do not want the shampoo to be doing much of its job close to the ends of your hair; instead, you want the shampoo to clean your scalp and remove any excessive sebum accumulation on the segment of the shaft closest to the scalp. This same issue of overaccumulation occurs with hair products too; hair products have a tendency to accumulate on the base of the hair shaft especially when applied incorrectly, which makes the use of hair products as part of the styling stage a tricky thing.

Shampoos are powerful cleaning agents, so bear that in mind when using them as improperly-used shampoo will dry out your moisturised and sebuminised mane in an instant. In fact, one of the main causes for the abundance of dead rats is precisely using too much shampoo and thus continually robbing one's locks from the much-needed scalp sebum!


## The optimal shampooing frequency

Now that you know the optimal shampooing method, it is time to learn how to find out your optimal shampooing frequency, which is just as important as how you go about applying the shampoo. Your shampooing frequency is central to your hair-grooming routine, and the rest of secondary actions in all stages of your hair-grooming routine will be dependent on your shampooing frequency.

As you know, shampoos are great at stripping away everything from your hair, including your own secreted sebum. You also know that sebum is imperative for the health and looks of your Is, Ss, Es or Zs and that, without this precious oil, your mane will not look its best. The question now arises, if shampoos are such powerful cleaning agents, how frequently should I use them then? Well, the answer is a bit more complicated than giving you a fixed number since shampooing frequency is quite individual and requires some trial and error to find out; however, daily use of shampoo is, in 99% of cases, not optimal or needed.

It is imperative for you to find out your optimal shampooing frequency so as to sport the best-looking hair because an optimal shampooing frequency strives for sebum harmony: you don't remove sebum too frequently, nor do you encourage too much of its accumulation. Moreover, it is not only excess sebum that needs to be removed but also any hairstyling products (e.g. hair gel) that you may use and that too need to be removed. Thus, the need for your hair to be cleaned daily calls for you to strive to find out your specific and optimal shampooing frequency with the knowledge and guidelines that are to follow. What's more is that finding out one's optimal shampooing frequency is actually a smooth and drama-free experience.

Before we dig into the whole finding out of your optimal shampooing frequency, I'd like to first put a full stop here and quickly tell you in the next 2 paragraphs about something that may very well go against what you thought was correct shampooing wisdom. Remember, to be able to sport your best hair, you must know not only the whats and hows of your hair but also the whys.

Not shampooing your hair daily is neither wrong nor unhygienic. Your mane will not become a dirty, foul, stinking, awful-looking beast; on the contrary, it will look, smell and feel better. My personal experience and my experience advising other men in hair-grooming matters have proven that shampooing daily is not the optimal way to go about having great hair. Even women don't shampoo every day, and, while we men can get away with rocking the caveman look if need be, 99% of women don't fancy rocking awful and smelly hair, hence there's certainly a merit to not shampooing daily if you want to maximise your hair's potential.

Back in the '60s with the advent of the hippie movement, shampoos were cunningly marketed by the big hair-care companies as bottled solutions for having clean and pure hair, or, in other words, you would not be a hippie if you shampooed your hair. Essentially, the more you shampooed, the less of a hippie you were, and thus housewives would rush daily to the bathroom to wash any hippiness off their children and keep it away as if it were some sort of demonic force. The myth prevailed as it was successfully ingrained in consumers' minds, and shampooing daily is still seen as the proper and only method to keeping one's hair clean. In a, perhaps, demonic paradox too, the vast majority of men who have come to me with bad hair and seeking a solution for it had the same hair-grooming flaw in common: they all shampooed their hair daily. Cutting their shampooing frequency to lower than daily was the easiest and most convenient way to quickly fix their locks; needless to say, not shampooing daily does work and is far from demonic!

So, after the above interesting paragraphs refuting conventional shampooing dogma, the question still remains, what is the optimal shampooing frequency to use? The answer is, it depends!

The optimal shampooing frequency to use is highly individual and will vary from one male to another although just about all men benefit from shampooing anywhere from "every other day" to "once a week", and it is within this range that you have to find out your optimal frequency. Such disparity in frequency among males is because we all have different scalps, hair types, hair lengths, preferences and lives. These are the main factors influencing the optimal shampooing frequency in men:

- Sebum secretion: this is defined by your genetic makeup, and some men just secrete more sebum than others.

- Hair products: some types of hair products tend to leave quite a bit of residue on the hair strands and scalp, which means that shampooing frequency has to be a bit higher than if you weren't using these products. Waxes and styling creams are among the heaviest residue-leaving hair products.

- Exposure to the environment: if you move around environments that encourage nasty stuff to stick to your hair (e.g. bars where people smoke, or you spend a lot of time outdoors), you should then schedule a shampooing session after each given exposure.

- Hair type: the curlier the hair type, the better it will fare with a lower shampooing frequency. Coiled and kinky hair types have the highest predisposition to dryness and not being fully sebuminised.

- Hair length: the longer your hair, the lower your shampooing frequency should be when compared to short hair.

- Preference: at the end of the day, if you prefer one frequency over the rest, your chances of adhering to it over the long term are higher.

The benefits that you will be obtaining from finding out your optimal shampooing frequency are:

- Hair will be less frizzy and dry.

- Shinier and more vigorous-looking hair.

- Less propensity for hair to tangle.

- Potentially-less scalp irritation from the harsh ingredients of shampoo (for those with sensitive skin).

- More convenience as you don't have to go through the whole shampooing ordeal every day (you will be cutting down time from your hair-grooming routine).

- Less of the unknown stuff that can be potentially absorbed by the scalp.

In other words, by finding out your optimal shampooing frequency, you will be obtaining the many bonuses that will pave the way for great-looking hair.

Now, on to the good stuff.

To find out what optimal shampooing frequency is best for you, you must ease off the shampooing slowly. If you shampoo daily, your scalp is literally hooked on the stuff so just stopping the shampoo altogether is going to make you go through some harsh shampoo withdrawals, which I can attest to being composed of your hair looking and feeling very greasy, with your scalp itching 24/7. You must drop your shampooing frequency slowly; take your time as, after all, your mane relationship is lifelong, so there is no need to rush its knowing.

For starters, I want you to start skipping the shampooing every other day, or what I call 1 on/1 off, with "on" being your shampooing day and "off" being your non-shampooing day. Thus, with 1 on/1 off, you shampoo one day, skip the shampoo the following day, and then you shampoo again on the third day. This is your starting point.

From there onwards, you will start adding an extra "off" day every 2 weeks until you find out your optimal shampooing frequency. However, in order to know when you have hit jackpot with your optimal frequency as you keep adding "off" days every 2 weeks, you should be striving to satisfy the following 5 indicators to shampooing frequency, which you will be reviewing at the end of each 2-week cycle per added "off" day. It will be once you satisfy these 5 indicators that you will have found out your optimal shampooing frequency:

1. Your hair looks fuller: you will notice that your hair will mysteriously start to look fuller and with more volume. This is completely normal and is a desired effect as your hair is starting to get optimal sebum coating and you are achieving sebum harmony.

2. Your hair will start to look less dry: again, sebum will now be allowed to optimally coat the hair strands, which means that your hair will look less dry.

3. Your hair will feel smoother upon running your fingers through it: dry hair feels hay-like whereas greasy hair feels hard to the touch (disgusting, even). Optimally-shampooed hair, on the other hand, feels smooth and light upon touching and feeling it, even when no hair products have been applied priorly.

4. Your scalp doesn't have an overaccumulation of sebum: an excess of sebum will manifest itself as small wax-like particles, which you will be able to notice in the mirror at first glance. You will know that you have lowered your shampooing frequency too much as these tiny particles are the first to show up when you are not shampooing with enough frequency.

5. <u>Your hair looks defined:</u> as you approach your optimal shampooing frequency, you will notice that your Is, Ss, Es or Zs will become more defined. Instead of looking like tumbleweed (dry hair) or looking plastered (greasy hair), your mane will look more eye-pleasing, and you will be able to see the enhanced definition of your hair in the mirror and so will others.

These listed 5 indicators are somewhat subjective. What is fuller to you, may not be as full to me, but the point remains; you will be noticing an increasing cosmetic benefit on your hair as it starts to look fuller, less dry, smoother, more defined, and no particles of overaccumulated sebum are to be seen on your mane. However, when in doubt, ask yourself, "would I let my hair look like this if I were to go on a first date with a hot chick?" That cue will tell you in an instant if you have currently hit your optimal shampooing frequency (married guys: instead, ask your ladies what they think of the gradual change in your hair, I don't want to incite you folks to think of any women other than your "one and only"!).

All right, so now that you know the aforementioned 5 indicators and what to look for when striving to find out your optimal shampooing frequency, this is how you will actually go about it:

- Hold the aforementioned initial 1 on/1 off shampooing frequency for 2 weeks. This is your starting frequency.

- Assess after those 2 weeks, and try to do the actual assessment when your hair has been fully dried and has no hairstyling products applied. Is your hair looking better? Have you satisfied the 5 indicators? If yes, you have found out your optimal frequency. If not, add another "off" day so that now you will be doing 1 on/2 off for the next 2 weeks. If you have found quite profound benefits with 1 on/1 off, you can still try 1 on/2 off if you fancy seeing whether you can get further cosmetic benefits or not.

- Reassess at the end of the 2 weeks with 1 on/2 off. Satisfied the 5 indicators? If yes, 1 on/2 off is for you. If not, add another "off" day for a 1 on/3 off schedule to be implemented for the next 2 weeks.

- After those 2 weeks of 1 on/3 off, reassess again and compare your results with the ideal results strived for in the 5 indicators. If you have satisfied them, then 1 on/3 off is your optimal frequency. If there is still some more room for improvement, add another "off" day for a new schedule of 1 on/4 off to be implemented for the next 2 weeks.

- And so on and so forth.

See the approach? You will continue to add an extra "off" day to your shampooing frequency until you satisfy the 5 indicators. Play it by the ear and don't make it complicated, you will already see results from 1 on/1 off, and, from there onwards, it is a matter of reassessing after each 2-week cycle per extra "off" day added. If you find out that, after the given 2 weeks of your newly-tried frequency, the 5 factors have regressed instead of continued to progress, then go back to your previous shampooing frequency as the one causing you to regress is not the optimal one at that time.

Do not panic if it takes you many weeks and you end up with a 1 on/7 off shampooing frequency or an even lower frequency of shampoo use; this is all completely normal, and your shampooing frequency will vary according to your unique set of circumstances as I explained earlier in this sub-subsection. Likewise, your shampooing frequency may have to be adjusted at times according to changes in your lifestyle. If you start going out more to bars where people smoke, or if you grow your hair longer (to give you 2 examples), you may need to alter your frequency. You should see your shampooing frequency as a readjustable process, which you will have to fine-tune as your hair-related circumstances change. Use the satisfying of the 5 indicators as your gauge to whether your current shampooing frequency is working or if you need to tweak it.

Since you will be experimenting with your shampooing frequency, it is imperative that you leave the rest of your hair-grooming routine intact during the timespan that it takes you to find out your optimal shampooing frequency. You will read later about the recommended hair-grooming routine to use, but, essentially, the routine that you will be using during this timespan is based on having a fixed set of secondary actions for your shampooing days and a fixed set of secondary actions for your non-shampooing days. Ergo, due to your shampooing frequency being central to your hair-grooming routine, it is best that you stick to a generic hair-grooming routine while you find out your optimal shampooing frequency for the first time.

Your optimal shampooing frequency is not static, and once you have found it out, you can modify it in the future whenever you notice that the 5 indicators are starting to take a hit due to external factors. Having said that, you now have the template and knowledge to find out (initially) and modify (later) your shampooing frequency as needed so that you are always using an optimal frequency, this being in itself a key element in achieving and maintaining great-looking hair for the rest of your life.

## The Sebum Coating method

Just because you will not be shampooing on some days, it doesn't mean that you should stop cleaning your hair altogether! On your non-shampooing days (i.e. "off" days), you will still go about your hair-grooming routine, soaking your hair with running water and then cleaning, conditioning and styling your mane. It will be on these "off" days that you will be doing the Sebum Coating method; do not be put off by the name because, just like with the optimal shampooing method, the Sebum Coating method is a convenient and fast method to getting your hair looking the part.

The Sebum Coating method consists of using your fingers to spread the scalp sebum across the whole length of the hair strands (i.e. sebuminise) so as to manually aid your locks in getting coated with this precious endogenous oil. This sebuminising method is performed on the days that you do not shampoo as these are the days when your secreted sebum is not removed by the shampoo. Moreover, the Sebum Coating method acts as a mild hair cleaner, removing any accumulated dust or mild residue from hair products as your fingers manually remove dirt through mechanical friction. Thus, the action of the Sebum Coating method is two-fold: to condition the hair by spreading the scalp sebum and to clean the hair via mechanical friction from the manual spreading motion. By doing the Sebum Coating method, you will be be keeping your hair conditioned and dirt free on your "off" days.

To do the Sebum Coating method, you need to completely soak your hair in water as if you were going to shampoo and then run your fingers gently through several hair locks at a time, with the finger-running motion starting from the base of the grabbed locks (scalp) and running to the very end of their length (tip). You run your fingers through the set of grabbed locks as water runs on it, and you only run your fingers through each set of locks once. The most efficient way to run your fingers is to pinch the thumb, index and middle fingers against the base of the locks and then move the fingers smoothly through the locks' length all the way to the tip.

Remember those 6 scalp segments that you will be using to apply the shampoo on your shampooing days (forehead, centre, both sides, vertex and nape)? Use the same pairing of segments, and simultaneously grab sets of hair locks from each segment at a time. Aim to grab as much hair as you can in about 1-inch-wide sets; typically, you will grab 3 to 10 hair locks in each 1-inch-wide set (depending on how thick your locks are naturally), and you can use wider sets or go lock by lock if you want to spend more time doing the Sebum Coating method (remember, a lock is nothing more than a group of hair strands growing next to each other and in the same direction). Just run your fingers once through each set of grouped locks, and then move on to the next set. Make sure that water is running on the set of hair locks that you are working on as you run your fingers, with the water being of a lukewarm temperature (not too hot, not too cold). Run your fingers fast and smoothly, avoiding any pulling of the locks; you are merely trying to spread a thin film of oil from the base of the locks to their tips, so there is no hair pulling involved here.

The point of the Sebum Coating method is to not only clean the hair but to also mobilise and spread the secreted scalp sebum with the help of your fingers so that the sebum can then coat the whole length of the hair strands. Since sebum is secreted by the sebaceous glands continuously and due to the tendency of sebum to stay close to the scalp in curly hair, this oily substance needs your help so as to travel across the entire length of the hair strands. Get your fingers working with the explained motion; you will even sometimes feel the sebum in your fingertips as you do the Sebum Coating method. Sebum is somewhat greasy yet odourless and clear, unless it has accumulated excessively as then it will resemble wax, and it will mean that you still haven't achieved your optimal shampooing frequency.

Overall, the Sebum Coating method will take you a maximum of 2 minutes to implement on all of your hair, less time once you master it. Remember, you only run your fingers once per set of hair locks, and you do it smoothly and fast; if the Sebum Coating method is taking you more than 2 minutes to complete, then aim to grab wider sets of locks. You can do the Sebum Coating method as frequently as you want although, as a bare minimum, you must implement it on your non-shampooing days for your first cleaning stage. If you are still unsure about what constitutes a lock of hair and how it relates to the Sebum Coating method, refer to Question 12 of Chapter 9 "Questions & Answers: The Miscellaneous Stuff You Will Ask Yourself".

Since the Sebum Coating method acts as a cleaning and conditioning agent, on your non-shampooing days the Sebum Coating method can also be used to substitute a conditioner for the second stage (conditioning) of your hair-grooming routine. What's more is that the actual action of the Sebum Coating method in the first stage as a hair cleaner already conditions the hair as the fingers spread the sebum, so there's no need to repeat the Sebum Coating method a second time for the conditioning stage. In other words, on your non-shampooing days, you can fuse both the first and second stages of your hair-grooming routine by just performing the Sebum Coating method and then moving on to the third styling stage.

The Sebum Coating method can also be performed on shampooing days if you so prefer. In this instance, the Sebum Coating method would be done prior to shampooing, meaning that the Sebum Coating method would the first secondary action of your hair-grooming routine on the given shampooing day. The biggest benefit of doing the Sebum Coating method before shampooing is that you will enhance the hair-cleaning action of the shampoo as you will have spread with your fingers any excess sebum that was found close to the scalp before cleaning the scalp with the shampoo. It is up to you if you want to do the Sebum Coating method on your shampooing days, but you certainly need to do the Sebum Coating method on your non-shampooing days for your first cleaning stage.

The Sebum Coating method is extremely useful, so do not skip it! With this method, you will encourage the optimal sebum coating of your mane while cleaning the hair, and you will be noticing your hair looking smoother, shinier and more defined once you get good at it.

## A shampooing note on hair types and hair length

As you can see in the next table (Figure 20), shampooing frequency typically differs according to hair type and hair length although the following frequencies in the table are just guidelines, and you may require a specific shampooing frequency that differs from what is typical for your hair type and given hair length.

Figure 20 – Typical shampooing frequency per hair type and extended length category
(High= 1 on/1 off, Very low= 1 on/7 off)

| | HAIR TYPES | | | |
|---|---|---|---|---|
| | *Straight* | *Wavy* | *Coiled* | *Kinky* |
| Near-shaved | High | High | Medium | Medium |
| Short | High | Moderate | Moderate | Low |
| Medium | High | Moderate | Low | Low |
| Long | Moderate | Low | Low | Very low |

As a rule of thumb, the curlier you hair type is, the lower the shampooing frequency that you will use because Es and Zs have a bigger issue than Is and Ss in getting coated optimally with sebum. Likewise, the curlier the hair type, the higher the predisposition to dryness, which means that shampoo should be used infrequently and the Sebum Coating method should be emphasised on every non-shampooing day to ensure the daily cleaning of one's hair while providing extra conditioning to the hair strands with the spread sebum.

When it comes to hair length, for every incremental length category that you grow your hair to (e.g. from short to medium), you should reduce your shampooing frequency by adding 1 extra "off" day, whatever your already established shampooing frequency may be. And the reverse goes for cutting your hair and going down in length category (e.g. from medium to short): you will increase your shampooing frequency by removing 1 "off" day per length category gone down to.

For example, say you followed the method to working out your optimal shampooing frequency for your 0.5-inch wavy hair (short-length category), and it turns out that a 1 on/2 off is the optimal frequency for you at that hair length. You then decide to grow your hair to 3 inches (medium length), and continue with your 1 on/2 off shampooing frequency right until your hair reaches the medium-length category (2-inch mark); you would then automatically add 1 extra "off" day to your current shampooing frequency, hence decreasing your shampooing frequency to 1 on/3 off as your waves have grown past the 2-inch mark. If, after some months, you decide to cut your hair and go from a medium length to a short length, then you would automatically remove 1 "off" day from your then-current 1 on/3 off to have a new shampooing frequency of

1 on/2 off as your hair has been cut to a short length (i.e. gone down 1 length category).

The reason behind decreasing your shampooing frequency as your hair grows is because the longer your hair is, the harder it is for your hair strands to get coated with sebum. Once your hair grows to a medium length and beyond, you need to pay special attention to how your hair is coated with sebum as optimal sebum coating is key to maintaining a great-looking mane. You must really get good at the Sebum Coating method and think of cleaning your hair as the first stage in your hair-grooming routine; a cleaning stage that is made of 3 equally important elements: shampooing method, shampooing frequency and the Sebum Coating method.

Of course, the above rules of thumbs are just that, rules of thumb; they are there to serve you as guidelines to fast-tracking the finding out of your specific shampooing frequency, the latter being an element of your hair-grooming routine that will not only vary according to your hair type and your hair length but that will also vary according to the unique set of circumstances that you find yourself in during different periods of your lifetime.

## A shampooing note on when your hair has too much residue

Over time, too much residue (i.e. buildup) from hairstyling products (and even sebum) may accumulate on your hair and both shampooing and the Sebum Coating method may not be enough to fully remove the accumulated residue. This typically occurs in cases where you have been using hairstyling products erroneously for too long. As you will learn further on in the section of this chapter that is dedicated to the styling stage of your hair grooming, you must apply your hairstyling products in a particular smart manner; otherwise, you run the risk of having layers of unremoved hairstyling products coating your hair shafts and drying the hair from the inside as no moisture from external sources is allowed into the shafts. The excess of unremoved hairstyling-product residue creates a noticeable effect by which your hair will feel heavy, greasy, hay-like and will loose its natural defined shape.

Through the No Shampoo method and your hair-grooming routine, you will be routinely cleaning the hair with great efficiency and effectiveness. However, you are not always guaranteed to be cleaning your hair optimally or to be applying the hairstyling products correctly, especially as you begin your journey to great-looking and convenient hair, and unremoved hairstyling products may start to pile up in your hair. Thus, it is in such scenarios where residue in your hair is not being responsive to your hair grooming that you can insert a special type of shampoo: a clarifying shampoo. This type of shampoo is quite similar to conventional shampoos except clarifying shampoos offer a stronger hair-cleaning functionality, meaning they are powerful shampoos and should not be used often (i.e. with a lesser frequency than your conventional shampoo). Clarifying shampoos are best used only for these scenarios in which you need to remove the piled-up sebum/product residue; clarifying shampoos are not to otherwise replace the use of your regular shampoo for your shampooing schedule.

Once you're coasting along with your newly-found optimal shampooing frequency, you may, at times, find your hair coated in an excess of residue caused by specific hair-grooming mistakes you've done as you're still new to the workings of the hair-equation system (e.g. a common mistake is using too much hairstyling product every day for weeks at a time); it is thus in these scenarios that you can use a clarifying shampoo to remove this unwanted buildup of residue. Likewise, you can use a clarifying shampoo right at the end of the period covering the finding out of your optimal shampooing frequency; once you have found out such essential frequency of shampoo use, then use a clarifying shampoo and start afresh your now worked-out optimal shampooing frequency with an uberly-cleaned scalp and locks.

Contrary to the shampoo application for the No Shampoo method, the clarifying shampoo should be allowed on all of your hair's length, not just on the scalp and segment of the hair strands closest to the scalp, for the goal is to remove absolutely everything that is coating your hair (whether good or bad) regardless of location. When you find your hair coated in a permanent layer of hairstyling products that is unresponsive to your usual shampooing and Sebum Coating method, then schedule a clarifying shampoo session as soon as possible and treat the session as that of a shampooing day (i.e. follow with a normal conditioner).

Resume your usual shampooing frequency after the clarifying-shampoo session; that is, treat the day after your clarifying-shampoo session as if you had used your usual conventional shampoo the day before instead of the clarifying shampoo, and the next shampooing day is to be performed with your usual shampoo.

## A note on the different types of shampoo

If you start browsing around for a shampoo, you will notice that quite a few shampoos make some very wild, and at times Mickey-Mouse, claims. Furthermore, you will quite likely encounter shampoos that claim to be for a specific "purpose" or of a specific "type". The reality is that the vast majority of shampoos simply play around with the percentage of a certain type of hair-cleaning ingredients (sulfate-type ingredients that acts as detergents) in the formula; thus, by lowering or increasing the hair-cleaning potency of the shampoo itself, hair-care companies can then come up with a range of shampoos and cater to specific hair-related issues. I will talk all about the hair-cleaning ingredients commonly used in shampoos in Question 7 of Chapter 9 "Questions & Answers: The Miscellaneous Stuff You Will Ask Yourself" although you don't need to flick forward to that chapter yet, for what you are going to be reading now will be explained as it goes.

Unfortunately, the hair-care industry is as regulated as Moscow's strip-club scene, which means that hair-care companies can and do get away with making plenty of wild claims and formulating products with exotic ingredients that are either suspect of not working or downright just don't work as advertised. Hair-care companies can make some hilariously-deceiving claims and get away with it so long as the ingredients added to the product are safe to use and have an iota of relevance to the advertised claim.

Fortunately, through the efforts of consumer groups and watchdog groups, hair-care companies have been called out for products that were unethically targeted and that were purposely made with claims that were bordering absolute lies; as a result, hair-care companies have gradually lowered the tone of their products' advertised claims over the last decade. All of this Mickey-Mouse nonsense is why I urge you to keep it simple when it comes to using shampoos and any other hair products because going back to the basics and keeping it minimal at the beginning is very important if you want to succeed in your hair-optimising journey.

Continuing from the above, the different "types" of shampoo do usually have other ingredients not found in conventional shampoos and that are inserted in the shampoos' formula in the hopes of providing an added specificity. The thing is, the different types of shampoo currently available are targeted for conditions and hair problems that you yourself will not be suffering from via the optimising of your hair-management equation (and the use of a conventional shampoo!). However, I feel that you should at least be aware of the different types of shampoo available in case you get lost in the nomenclature of modern-day shampoos; overall, there are 7 types of shampoo and they are:

- Regular shampoo

- Oil-removing shampoo

- Clarifying shampoo

- Moisturising shampoo

- Volumising shampoo

- Chelating shampoo

- Dandruff shampoo

## Regular shampoo

"Regular" shampoo can go by other names such as "normal shampoo", "daily shampoo" or "gentle shampoo", or it can simply not have any extra word added before "shampoo". Regular shampoos are what I refer to as "conventional shampoos" in this book and are the type of shampoo to use when finding out your shampooing frequency. In this book, any time that I refer to shampoo without specifying its actual type, I will be referring to regular shampoo.

Regular shampoos contain commonly-added sulfate-type ingredients plus some other ingredients that most of the time simply add to the hype of the shampoo. In the ingredient label of a regular shampoo, look for the sulfate-type ingredients discussed in Question 7 of Chapter 9 "Questions & Answers: The Miscellaneous Stuff You Will Ask Yourself" when you choose your shampoo for the finding out of your optimal shampooing frequency, and don't overcomplicate your life with minutiae.

## Oil-removing shampoo

"Oil-removing" shampoos are more potent than regular shampoos and are intended for chronically-oily scalps; their increased potency is achieved by either increasing the percentage of the hair-cleaning ingredients in the formula or by adding more hair-cleaning ingredients. Typically, you will see the ingredient "cocamidopropyl betaine" together with sulfate-type ingredients in the label of oil-removing shampoos: cocamidopropyl betaine is a surfactant ingredient and enhances the overall hair-cleaning effect of sulfate-type ingredients. Mind you, regular shampoos may also contain cocamidopropyl betaine, but oil-removing shampoos have more of it.

Oil-removing shampoos are normally advertised for oily hair and tend to be labelled as "shampoo for oily hair" or imply in the label that the shampoo is for men with oily scalps or hair. However, and this is a big however, "oily hair" is a condition suffered by men who do not wisely look after their hair (unlike you), which is why the different types of shampoo that differ from regular shampoos (including this one) are mostly irrelevant to you.

Having said the above, you may, though, use this product as your "regular shampoo" (i.e. to use on your "on" days) if you so wish to, but only do this after having found out your optimal shampooing frequency with a regular shampoo. And, of course, do adapt your shampooing frequency to this change in shampoo type.

## Clarifying shampoo

As you have learnt in the previous subsection, "clarifying" shampoos are to be used when an excessive buildup of sebum and/or hairstyling products occurs over time. Clarifying shampoos are great at removing the buildup from the 2 aforementioned sources of residue, and the cleaning magic of clarifying shampoos occurs via the inclusion (in the formula) of the highest concentration of hair-cleaning agents such as sulfate-type ingredients, cocamidopropyl betaine (and chemically-related ingredients) and also acidic agents such as acetic acid or citric acid.

Clarifying shampoos are normally advertised as such, although they can go by other shampoo names that imply a very strong hair-cleaning action; some words used for their advertising include "anti-residue", "anti-scaling" and "detoxifying". In any case, always refer to the ingredient list and look for the aforementioned hair-cleaning ingredients. In the case that the shampoo advertised as "clarifying" doesn't contain cocamidopropyl betaine (or a chemically-related ingredient) and an acidic agent, then ensure that the sulfate-type ingredients included in the formula are right at the top (or beginning) of the ingredient list. To understand how the listing of ingredients works, refer to Question 8 of Chapter 9.

Overall, clarifying shampoos are the super-charged version of regular shampoos and are thus to be used only when the buildup of residue is not responding any more to your hair-grooming efforts and shampooing frequency. Treat your scheduled clarifying-shampoo session as an "on" day, following the rinsing of the clarifying shampoo with a normal conditioner. The next day, continue with your normal shampooing frequency as if you had used your regular shampoo instead of the clarifying shampoo the day before.

## Moisturising shampoo

"Moisturising" shampoos are a type of shampoo that claims to add moisture to the hair strands and help to condition the hair, thus moisturising shampoos can also be found labelled as "nourishing shampoos". The ingredient list of moisturising shampoos will contain commonly-added hair-cleaning ingredients plus hair-conditioning ingredients that can range from the ingredients commonly added to conditioners (I also talk about these ingredients in Question 7 of Chapter 9) to some exotic ingredients that may or may not work as claimed.

Personally, I've yet to find a moisturising shampoo that works, for these shampoos tend to sacrifice part of their hair-cleaning strength for their purported moisturising action, for which the latter is also not as strong as the conditioning action of conditioners themselves; thus, you're left with a mediocre product most of the time that neither cleans well enough nor conditions the hair sufficiently. Because this type of shampoo claims to work on dry hair, it will not really relate to your case as dry hair is an issue that is already factored into the workings of the hair-management equation, which then adds further emphasis to the irrelevance of moisturising shampoos when it comes to your specific hair case.

In any case, if you want to experiment with moisturising shampoos, by all means, do so, but only after you've worked out your optimal shampooing frequency with a regular shampoo. Lastly, moisturising shampoos do certainly have their place in the hair-care industry as they can somewhat make up for a lack of conditioning in the erratic hair grooming of men who do not follow a proper hair-grooming method such as the one you are learning with my hair-equation system.

## Volumising shampoo

"Volumising" shampoos work on the premise of adding thickness to otherwise thin hair caused by one's genetic makeup or by male pattern baldness (MPB), thus volumising shampoos are also known as "thickening shampoos". The purported thickening hair effect occurs via the temporary swelling of the shaft together with the depositing of ingredients on the cuticle. The specific volumising ingredients commonly added to volumising shampoos include panthenol (pro-vitamin B5) and protein-derived proteins such as wheat protein, rice protein and silk protein. Mind you, you may find these ingredients added to certain brands of other types of shampoo, but the aforementioned ingredients are what cause volumising shampoos to work.

Volumising shampoos only work their intended thickening effect temporarily (until you clean your hair again), and these shampoos leave quite some residue behind, which means that your shampooing frequency will very likely increase upon using volumising shampoos. Furthermore, don't think of volumising shampoos as magic shampoos that will give you luscious, uber-thick locks; most volumising shampoos either give a slightly thickening effect to your hair or don't do anything at all.

If you're worried about your hair thinning, then I recommend you to see a dermatologist and get on minoxidil if you are suffering from MPB; minoxidil is a substance that has a noticeable positive effect on MPB, both for regrowing hair and for thickening existing hair strands. Using a volumising shampoo together with minoxidil is quite a commonly-used regimen for the management of MPB.

## Chelating shampoo

A chelating shampoo is a type of shampoo that claims to remove the gradual buildup of minerals on your hair that may not be fully removed with your regular shampoo.

A chelating shampoo can be of use to you if you live in an area with hard water or if you are constantly in the swimming pool (e.g. you're are a competitive swimmer and train in the pool several days per week). The best way to remove the buildup of minerals from frequent, long-term exposure to hard water or swimming-pool water is to schedule a shampooing session with a chelating shampoo.

The ingredients used in chelating shampoos are chelating agents, which bond to the minerals that still remain on your hair and thus allow for the complete removal of the mineral buildup from the hair. The main chelating agents used in chelating shampoos are EDTA (ethylenediaminetetraacetic acid) and any of its salt forms as well as sodium citrate. A chelating shampoo will be advertised as "chelating" and will sometimes be advertised as both clarifying and chelating. Be aware that EDTA is also used in regular shampoos to stabilise the shampoo under a hard-water scenario and allow for the shampoo to do its hair-cleaning job, which is why, even though you may live in a hard-water area, you may still not need a chelating shampoo by itself. Having short or medium-length hair and getting your hair trimmed frequently further decreases any need for a chelating shampoo.

If you are exposed to the 2 aforementioned sources of mineral buildup, then you may benefit from using a chelating shampoo, especially if your hair has lost its shine and definition and also feels heavy despite no changes in your hair-grooming routine or hair-care strategy. The frequency of use of a chelating shampoo should be once a month, though you can play with a slightly-higher (or lower) frequency depending on the severity of your exposure. Use the chelating shampoo on your shampooing day, replacing your regular shampoo with this type of shampoo for that specific day. Follow the chelating shampoo with a conditioner and continue with your usual shampooing schedule and frequency the next day.

**Dandruff shampoo**

Dandruff shampoos contain certain active ingredients that are aimed at controlling the higher-than-normal shedding of dead skin cells from the scalp that occurs in certain people; this excessive shedding of dead skin cells being what is commonly referred to as "dandruff" when the excessive shedding occurs in the scalp. There is no true cure for dandruff, and dandruff shampoos help in managing dandruff when it is notoriously at its worst (e.g. winter time). Dandruff shampoos can be used regularly or on and off depending on how bad your dandruff is; furthermore, dandruff shampoos must be used as directed in the product's instructions and the vast majority of dandruff shampoos should not replace your regular shampoo (i.e. use dandruff shampoos while maintaining your regular-shampoo use).

The actual active ingredients found in dandruff shampoos will vary, and you can find a wide range of dandruff shampoos over the counter as well as through prescription. I will cover below the range of over-the-counter dandruff shampoos available because medical shampoos have to be prescribed by a dermatologist; having said this, most medical shampoos are also found as over-the-counter dandruff shampoos but with lowered concentrations of the active ingredients that would otherwise be found in the respective medical version. Lastly, in terms of dandruff shampoos, what's sold over the counter and what's only sold with a prescription will also vary according to the country, so always check with your pharmacist if you decide to buy a dandruff shampoo over the counter.

For what is worth, whether you decide to treat your dandruff case with an over-the-counter dandruff shampoo or a medical dandruff shampoo, it's in your interest to always see a dermatologist if your dandruff is getting out of hand because treating your dandruff case with over-the-counter shampoos may be masking the root (no pun intended) of your scalp issue, which you may have mistaken for dandruff.

Below are the active ingredients typically found in over-the-counter dandruff shampoos; these ingredients are proven to help in the management of dandruff when found in combination or alone in dandruff shampoos and when used as indicated and directed by the product's instructions or by your dermatologist:

- Zinc pyrithione: this is an ingredient that is both antifungal and antibacterial, and which helps to tame the Malassezia globosa fungus that is found in the scalp; this fungus can cause inflammation of the scalp and thus an increased cell turnover and increased shedding of dead skin cells (i.e. dandruff). Dandruff shampoos that contain zinc pyrithione as the sole dandruff-treating active ingredient are the only type of dandruff shampoo that can be used as regular shampoos for the "on" days of your shampooing frequency (provided that the zinc-pyrithione dandruff shampoo also contains the same hair-cleaning ingredients found in regular shampoos). Furthermore, zinc pyrithione can also

*(follows from previous page)*

be found combined with any of the other anti-dandruff ingredients in a dandruff shampoo.

- Coal tar: this is an ingredient that is a byproduct of the coal-manufacturing process and that helps to tame dandruff by decreasing the amount of dead-skin-cell production in your scalp. Incidentally, paracetamol (aka acetaminophen) is derived from coal tar too.

- Salicylic acid: this ingredient is found in dandruff shampoos that are usually called "scalp-scrubbing shampoos" or "exfoliating shampoos". Shampoos containing salicylic acid will remove the dead skin cells that have excessively accumulated on your scalp, but these specific shampoos may also leave your scalp (and hair) completely dry by also removing your sebum. You can think of salicylic-acid-based shampoos for the treatment of dandruff as the equivalent of clarifying shampoos for the removal of sebum/hairstyling-product residue.

- Selenium sulfide: this ingredient is believed to control both cell turnover and the Malassezia globosa fungus in the scalp. Selenium sulfide is reported to increase oiliness of the scalp in some users and can also discolour blonde, grey and dyed hair.

- Ketoconazole: this ingredient is a broad-spectrum antifungal agent that not only works on the Malassezia globosa fungus but is also active against other fungi and yeast that can cause further scalp disorders and hair loss. Several dandruff shampoos containing ketoconazole are commercially available and are also advertised to treat hair loss (evidence for the latter condition is not as solid as the evidence found for the treatment of dandruff).

- Ciclopirox olamine: this ingredient is also an antifungal agent although its precise mechanism of action for the treatment of dandruff is poorly understood (it is believed to work differently to ketoconazole though). If you find that ketoconazole as an antifungal is not correcting your dandruff, then ciclopirox olamine is a good antifungal alternative.

- <u>Neem and tea-tree oil:</u> these 2 tree-derived substances have antifungal properties and both of them have been shown to be effective against dandruff. More so, they can potentially aid in hair loss exacerbated by scalp fungi and yeast; tea-tree oil has some good anecdotal evidence vouching for its effectiveness to treat male pattern baldness when used in combination with other hair-growing compounds as a regimen.

Since this subsection is notably large, I will list again the 7 types of shampoo that we have gone through in this subsection:

- Regular shampoo

- Oil-removing shampoo

- Clarifying shampoo

- Moisturising shampoo

- Volumising shampoo

- Chelating shampoo

- Dandruff shampoo

As you have been able to read in this whole subsection, most types of shampoo available are formulated to target a specific hair-related issue that you will not be experiencing upon optimising your hair-management equation. Because most males walk around with hair that is erratically cared for and that is groomed with no consistency or order, the different types of shampoo are thus formulated so as to solve a problem that is caused, more than anything else, by neglect. What's worse is that some of these special shampoos simply don't work as advertised or are advertised to produce dramatic results when all they yield are very-small benefits.

If you want to use a type of shampoo that is not of the regular type, you must only do so after having already found out your optimal shampooing frequency through the use of a regular shampoo. This is imperative because the different types of shampoo will impact your shampooing frequency and overall hair-grooming schedule in one way or another.

In the case of dandruff shampoos, incorporate their use together with your use of a regular shampoo. However, a zinc-pyrithione-based shampoo can replace your regular shampoo, both for the finding out of your shampooing frequency and as your go-to shampoo for your "on" days. If you are using a medical shampoo, you must consult your dermatologist prior to modifying your current shampooing schedule.

## **Second stage – Conditioning**

Conditioning is the second stage of your hair-grooming routine, and it is performed after you have rinsed the shampoo or implemented the Sebum Coating method. Your conditioning action is performed with a conditioner: a hair-grooming product that does its conditioning job by allowing the hair strands to retain moisture (i.e. prevents dryness) while providing gloss. Moreover, conditioners enhance the slip between locks and, overall, improve the manageability of one's mane. Thus, conditioners are great weapons for you to have in your hair-grooming arsenal because dryness is a big issue that wreaks havoc in every male's head of hair, and conditioners tackle this issue from the very root (no pun intended).

Your scalp already secretes an awesome conditioner: your own sebum. Unfortunately, sebum can't always do its job properly, and artificial conditioners provide an extra aid to your mane to make your locks look great. Now that you know how to make the most of your own natural conditioner via the Sebum Coating method, it is time to know how to use conditioners as these products will provide an extra advantage, on top of your own sebum, to make your mane awesome.

There are 2 types of conditioners that are of need to you: normal conditioners and leave-in conditioners. Normal conditioners need to be applied and left on your hair for 2 minutes after having cleaned the hair, and they are rinsed after the 2-minute count. On the other hand, leave-in conditioners are used when styling your mane in the third stage and are not rinsed or washed away until you clean your hair again. Incidentally, normal conditioners are used in the second stage of your hair grooming, and leave-in conditioners are used in the third stage within the same routine (i.e. leave-ins are used in the styling stage, not in the conditioning stage). However, both types of conditioners have the same main action: to condition the hair strands, and they can be used concomitantly on the same day.

Both types of conditioners are key in building great-looking hair, and you will benefit from them extensively if you use them the correct way. Conditioners are of special use to men with the curliest of hair types (coiled and kinky) because these hair types have the biggest issue with dryness and in getting coated with sebum, and because tangling of the hair strands is a very prominent issue the curlier one's hair is. However, both types of conditioners are of great use to all hair types, and you should have them in your hair-grooming arsenal regardless of your hair type.

## Normal conditioners

Normal conditioners are predominantly used on your shampooing days following the rinsing of the shampoo, although they can also be used on your non-shampooing days after the Sebum Coating method. Regarding their name, normal conditioners are simply labelled as "conditioners" or "rinse-out" conditioners by hair-care companies, but I prefer to call them "normal conditioners" in this book so as to avoid confusion with leave-in conditioners.

Normal conditioners are hair products that leave a thin film coating the hair strands in a similar way as to how sebum is intended to do. The thin film left by normal conditioners acts to seal in moisture into the hair strands while smoothing out the cuticle of the hair shaft, which translates into a cosmetic benefit to your mane. Normal conditioners also have a lubricating effect, meaning that they are great tools to keep your locks free of tangles. Lastly, normal conditioners provide gloss (i.e. make the hair shinier) and ultimately allow you to manage your hair with more ease.

You should use a normal conditioner straight after you rinse the shampoo from your hair. Pour the conditioner on your palms and rub them together so as to spread the conditioner on the fingers of both your hands, leaving a thick film of conditioner coating the fingers. Then, use your fingers to apply the conditioner to all of your hair, aiming to coat the hair strands with a film of conditioner from mid-length to the tips. What you have just read is very important: do not apply the conditioner to the segment of the hair strands close to the scalp or on the scalp itself (i.e. the reverse of the shampoo application).

With regards to hair dryness, the problem lies in the area between the mid-length and the tip of the hair shaft as this is the segment of the hair that most commonly doesn't get enough moisture retention. While the Sebum Coating method will maximise the spread of sebum across the length of the hair strands, it is only normal that a good chunk of the sebum will remain closest to where it is secreted from: the scalp. Thus, you must emphasise the application of the conditioner from mid-length all the way up to the tip of the hair for that's where the conditioner is most needed (i.e. where it will aid in retaining moisture).

Use plenty of normal conditioner and generously, but be careful if you have short-length hair as it is easy to get the conditioner on your scalp unintentionally. After applying it to your hair, leave the conditioner on without rinsing for 2 minutes while you continue grooming and cleaning the rest of your body in the shower. Once the 2 minutes are over, rinse the conditioner with running water, making sure that the washed-away conditioner doesn't go in your eyes because, just like with shampoo, you don't want the stuff near your eyes. About 30 seconds is more than enough to wash away all the conditioner from your hair.

Again, normal conditioners are used in the second stage of your shampooing days and following the rinsing of the shampoo. However, you can also use normal conditioners on the days that you do not shampoo (i.e. non-shampooing days) but only after the Sebum Coating method, not before. Essentially, your own secreted sebum is your de facto conditioner on your non-shampooing days, yet you can also add extra conditioning on these "off" days by using a normal conditioner after the Sebum Coating method.

Indeed, while the Sebum Coating method is more than enough for your conditioning action on your non-shampooing days, occasionally using normal conditioners on your "off" days can be beneficial especially for those men with coiled and kinky hair as well as for those men with long hair. The good thing is that using a very high frequency of normal conditioner use (e.g. daily) will not have much of a negative impact on your mane as opposed to using a too-high shampooing frequency (e.g. daily), so feel free to introduce normal conditioners on your "off" days if you are keen to experiment. A good starting point that I have used in the past is to introduce normal conditioners on 50% of my non-shampooing days, but you can play around with higher percentages without fearing a dead rat. In any case, do remember that normal conditioners must be used on your shampooing days, and any further use on your "off" days will be subject to trial and error as well as personal preference.

## Leave-in conditioners

Leave-in conditioners work as normal conditioners and have the same purpose. The difference is that leave-ins are left on the hair and can also be used to style one's hair as a hairstyling product. Unlike the normal variety, you don't apply the leave-in conditioner in the shower, and you don't rinse it either. You get out of the shower; you dry your hair so that it is left in a damp state, and you then apply the leave-in conditioner to your hair as you work your chosen hairstyle. Consequently, leave-ins are used in the third styling stage and not in the second conditioning stage despite leave-ins having a main conditioning action like normal conditioners have.

To use a leave-in conditioner, the same application rule goes as with normal conditioners: do not get the leave-in anywhere near the scalp, only apply from mid-length to the tip of the hair. Put some in your fingers and work your way through your locks to coat the hair with a film of leave-in conditioner, then proceeding to style your mane. Some leave-in conditioners also come in handy sprays; yet, no matter what their packaging form is, the main action of a leave-in conditioner is to condition the hair, and all leave-ins are not to be rinsed and can be used as products to style the hair.

Leave-in conditioners should ideally be used for your styling stage on your non-shampooing days after the Sebum Coating method, although they can also be used daily and without regard to your shampooing frequency, or you can use them whenever you desire as you play around with their frequency of use. They are of special value once your hair has reached a medium length, and leave-ins can be used in conjunction with other hairstyling products (leave-in conditioner first, then the other product) or used alone to style the hair. And as with normal conditioners, don't get the stuff on the scalp or in your eyes!

## Conditioners, the Sebum Coating method and putting it all together

Normal and leave-in conditioners are great, but the Sebum Coating method is just as great. The 3 used together, however, works like magic.

The Sebum Coating method has an important hair-conditioning action apart from its also important hair-cleaning action, hence the Sebum Coating method satisfies the second conditioning stage of your hair-grooming routine. The Sebum Coating method fuses both first and second stages on your non-shampooing days, and it allows you to go straight to the third stage (i.e. styling) without having to use a normal conditioner as you'd otherwise do after your first stage on your shampooing days.

Normal conditioners are a must on your shampooing days. On your non-shampooing days, you can strictly soak your hair in water, do the Sebum Coating method and then get out of the shower to style your mane, skipping the normal conditioner. However, on your shampooing days, you must use a normal conditioner after rinsing the shampoo; once you have applied and rinsed the normal conditioner, you can then move on to the third styling stage.

In addition to the above, you can also include a normal conditioner for your second stage on your non-shampooing days after the Sebum Coating method: a good starting point is to use a normal conditioner on 50% of your non-shampooing days. Some men with the curliest of hairs (i.e. kinky hair) may find out that they need to practically use normal conditioners every day without consideration to shampooing frequency and despite using the Sebum Coating method on their stipulated non-shampooing days.

Leave-in conditioners are very handy tools, and they can be used together with other hairstyling products (e.g. hair gel) to put your hair into a hairstyle. Leave-ins not only serve a conditioning purpose but they are also great hairstyling agents for those hairstyles in which hair doesn't need to be held in position. Leave-in conditioners can be used every day, and they are very easy to remove the next time that you clean your hair with a shampoo or the Sebum Coating method. Ergo, when you are really pressed for time on your non-shampooing days, you can jump in the shower, do the Sebum Coating method, then move to styling your hair with a leave-in conditioner and rush out the door with a moisturised and sebum-optimised head of Is, Ss, Es or Zs.

As a drastic measure, you can even skip using a leave-in conditioner on your non-shampooing days, but, ideally and so as to ensure the conditioning of your mane, you should use a leave-in conditioner on your non-shampooing days as part of the third styling stage and after the Sebum Coating method. Once your hair reaches a medium length though, you will tangibly discover that using a leave-in conditioner on just about every day is the best way to keep your mane looking great. As a matter of fact, you may find that only using a leave-in conditioner as your de facto hairstyling product is the best way forward to sport great-looking hair.

For what is worth, many men who come to me for hair advice are not only unaware of what hair conditioners actually are, but they also have a wrong perception or attitude towards these hair-grooming products. No, conditioners are not for girls; and, no, they will not require half of your morning to apply and use. As you have learnt in this section, both normal and leave-in conditioners are fundamental pieces of the conditioning action, and they are convenient and useful tools that will allow you to build your optimal hair-grooming routine and thus have you sporting the best-looking mane that you can possibly own.

## <u>Third stage – Styling</u>

Styling your hair is the third stage and final main action of your hair-grooming routine, and it involves the following secondary actions:

1. Using the right hairstyling agent (i.e. hairstyling product) to get your mane looking as you want it to look. A leave-in conditioner is included here as one of the hairstyling agents available to use.

2. Knowing what you want as a hairstyle, and putting your mane into one.

3. Taking your hair from wet to damp (i.e. dry your hair) so as to prepare it for styling.

While I will cover a wide array of hairstyles available to you in Chapter 6 "Giving Your Mane Its Shape: Hairstyles, Hair Accessories, Straightening Your Locks, Growing That Mane And Getting A Haircut", it is best that this styling section is dedicated to outlining the different hairstyling agents available to you as well as the essentials of styling your hair; it is only once you know these that you can truly make the most of any hairstyles you may so choose. You will read about the hairstyles recommended for each hair type in the sixth chapter so as to not have you overloaded with information in this chapter; thus, for now, let's us concentrate on the core of your styling stage.

Styling your mane is the last stage of the hair-grooming process (i.e. routine), and it is here where you can be a bit more casual and lax: hair that is properly moisturised will already look great without a true need to style it. So long as you use shampoos smartly, make the most of your own sebum and use conditioners appropriately, you will already have the grooming foundation for a great head of Is, Ss, Es or Zs. The styling puts the icing on the cake.

## Hairstyling agents

Unfortunately, many men make the mistake of looking at hairstyling agents (i.e. hairstyling products) as the fix to their hair dramas without even considering that the solution to their dead rats may rest elsewhere. To put it bluntly, to achieve your best hair, you must have the first 2 hair-grooming stages optimised before beginning to think about hairstyling agents and hairstyles to put your mane into.

Alright, now that I have emphasised the importance of the 2 previous hair-grooming stages, let's talk about hairstyling agents!

When it comes to styling your hair, you can go solo (i.e. no hairstyling agent), or you can use a hairstyling agent or a blend of several. Hairstyling "agents" only differ from hairstyling "products" in that agents include not only all hairstyling commercial products but also include natural oils and butters, the latter 2 not necessarily sold as hair products and which can be found in food stores. Thus, I prefer to use "agents" as a term to denote any product, commercial or not, that can be used to style your hair.

Overall, there are 8 main hairstyling agents that you can use to style your hair with:

1. Gel

2. Pomade

3. Wax

4. Mousse

5. Leave-in conditioner

6. Styling cream

7. Hair spray

8. Natural oils and butters

All of the aforementioned hairstyling agents differ in ingredients and functionality. What's more is that some are better suited to certain hair types. For example, men with straight hair and wavy hair tend to benefit from hair gels and waxes, whereas those with coiled hair and kinky hair tend to find leave-in conditioners, oils or going solo with an emphasis on the Sebum Coating method to be of greater benefit. You can find in Appendix XXVII, Appendix XXVIII and Appendix XIX a series of tables listing the most suitable hairstyling agents per each hair type and hair length. Don't worry about these tables for now though, they will be most useful once you have understood and grasped the knowledge of this whole chapter, so leave their studying for later.

With hairstyling agents, you will find that you will need to experiment a little to find out the one (or a blend of) that is best suited to you. While in this section you will learn the details and guidelines to each hairstyling agent and how useful each is to a specific hair type, trialling different hairstyling agents (and even brands within each agent) will be of benefit to you especially since, at the end of the day, personal preference is key in choosing and adhering to one's hair-grooming routine.

All of the 8 hairstyling agents are applied when you hair is damp, not wet or dry. That means that styling your mane as part of your hair-grooming routine normally occurs in the morning when you are done in the shower and then get out of the shower to take your hair from wet to damp (i.e. dry your hair). Never apply a hairstyling agent to your mane when the hair has fully dried and isn't damp; either apply the agent after you shower and the hair is damp, or quickly dampen your locks with water before applying your chosen hairstyling agent. Likewise, all these hairstyling agents are applied to your hair as you'd do with conditioners: from the hair strands' mid-length all the way to the tips, never close to the scalp (remember, shampoo is the only hair-grooming product that you use on your scalp).

Because you, as a modern male desiring convenient aesthetic hair, need to know what weapons you can have in your hair-grooming arsenal for mane awesomeness, I will now go through each hairstyling agent available as well as their pros and cons so that you can decide for yourself which to use and integrate into the third stage of what constitutes your hair-grooming routine. Do note, however, that hair-care companies sometimes innovate the formulation of one of their hairstyling agents, having the agent behave differently than what would otherwise be expected; so, in terms of expectations, always treat any new hairstyling agent that you buy with caution.

## Hair gel

Quite likely, you will already be familiar with hair gels. They come in a variety of "holds" (i.e. strengths), and they are great for straight and wavy hair ranging from short to medium length as hair gel is very useful to hold (secure in place) the hair in many hairstyles. Hair gel should be avoided by those with kinky hair although "light hold" hair gel can be used in small quantities to provide the finishing touches for this curliest of hair types.

Pros:

- Lasts the whole day.

- Holds hair in place; awesome for hairstyles requiring hair to remain fixed.

- Great for sculpting a hairstyle (best for Is and Ss, though).

- Wide variety of cool smells.

- Will define waves and coils.

Cons:

- Leaves residue on your hair.

- Can lead to tangling of your hair, especially if it is coiled or kinky.

- Will impede your locks from hanging fully loose.

- Strong-hold gel can make long hair look like nasty crunchy sticks.

## Hair pomade

Unlike hair gel, hair pomade doesn't dry fully, and it gives hair a shiny look. Hair pomade is best used on the straight, wavy and coiled hair types, ranging from short to medium length.

Pros:

- Lasts the whole day.

- Makes hair look slick.

- Makes hair shiny and glossy.

- Neutral smell.

- Will define waves and coils.

- Will help your hair hang down.

Cons:

- Difficult to remove, leaves some residue.

- Can make hair look greasy if you apply too much.

- Not the best hairstyling agent to hold hair in place.

## Hair wax

Hair waxes are the more solid version of pomades. They are better than pomades for holding hair in place, and they do not dry fully either. Wax works best on short to medium-length Is and Ss, and, unlike pomade, hair wax is a good option for hairstyles that encourage the defying of gravity.

Pros:

- Lasts the whole day.

- Works good for holding hair in place.

- Great for sculpting a hairstyle.

- Gives a shiny look.

- Will define wavy hair.

Cons:

- Difficult to remove, leaves lots of residue.

- Will make coiled and kinky hair look frizzy (use tiny amounts if you insist on using wax).

- Can leave hair looking greasy very fast if overdone.

- Needs some more application time as you must pay extra attention to not get the hair wax on your scalp.

- Not suitable for long-length Ss, Es or Zs.

## Hair mousse

Hair mousse is great for making your hair look more voluminous. It still holds the hair in place, yet it also adds a volumising element to your styling. It is best used on straight and wavy hair as these are the hair types that have the least natural volume of the 4 hair types, so hair mousse is a great tool for hairstyles aiming to style the hair with a big-volume emphasis. Hair mousse works the greatest on medium to long-length hair and can be used with a hair dryer to enhance the acquired extra hair volume (apply the hair mousse first, then use the hair dryer).

Pros:

- Works reasonably well to hold hair in place.

- Will add plenty of volume to your hair regardless of hair type.

- Will define the curly hair types (wavy, coiled and kinky).

- Works great for hairstyles requiring "puffing out" (volumising) and the use of a hair dryer.

- Easy to wash off.

- Will give a wet-look effect when combined with some hair spray.

- Unintentionally getting some on your scalp is not as bad as the rest of hairstyling agents.

Cons:

- Not great for sculpting hairstyles.

- Will not last the whole day if you are active (e.g. you spend time outdoors or in the gym).

- Will give the nasty "crunchy stick" look if you overdo it.

- Not the best hairstyling agent for short-length hair or kinky hair.

## Leave-in conditioner

Leave-in conditioners not only work as de facto normal conditioners but they also work as hairstyling agents to use if you want your hair to be hanging down and looking glossy. Leave-in conditioners are useful for all hair types and lengths, and they can be used alone as a hairstyling agent or together with other hairstyling agents. Leave-in conditioners are also a necessary item when your hair reaches a medium length regardless of your hair type. If you want to use a leave-in with other hairstyling agents, always apply the leave-in first.

Pros:

- Conditions and moisturises your hair like no other hairstyling agent.

- Great to use if you want your hair to hang down (best done in combination with a styling cream).

- Easy to remove.

- Doesn't dry excessively like hair gel does.

- Overdoing it will not make your hair freak out like hair gel or hairspray will do.

- Works great in combination with any other hairstyling agents especially hair gel and styling creams.

- Convenient; you can apply it quickly and be done in seconds.

- Will help define your Ss, Es and Zs.

- Provides ample slip to the hair strands, which will help in keeping your mane tangle free.

- Unintentionally getting some on your scalp is not as bad as with the rest of hairstyling agents.

Cons:

- Doesn't hold hair in place.

- Not good for sculpting a hairstyle.

- Not suitable for short-length hair as a standalone hairstyling agent, combine with another hairstyling agent for best aesthetic results if you have a short-length mane.

- Should be used daily with medium/long-length waves, coils or kinks (though its application is fast and convenient).

## Styling cream

A styling cream is a neater version of a pomade and is great for taming frizz and adding shine. Styling creams add weight to the hair, so they are very useful to weight down your Is, Ss, Es and Zs if you want them to hang down at lengths in which they still defy gravity in a natural/no hair-product state. All hair types benefit from styling creams although this hairstyling agent is particularly suited for coiled and kinky hair at medium lengths and longer especially if used to make these hair types hang down.

Pros:

- Great for defining waves, coils and kinks.

- Good at taming frizz and flyaway hairs.

- Adds shine with a wet-look effect.

- Adds weight to hair, which helps it to hang down at medium and long lengths.

Cons:

- Doesn't hold hair in place very well.

- Despite being lighter in residue than wax, it is still a nuisance to remove.

- Not optimal for short-length straight hair (instead, use hair gel, pomade or wax).

- Can make hair look greasy if overdone.

## Hair spray

Hair spray is used to harden your hair and hold it in place like no other. Hair spray can be used on any hair type, and it should be viewed as the finishing touch to secure your hair for those hairstyles or occasions in which you want to rock a certain look day long. When used with hair mousse, it can give a wet look too (apply the hair mousse first, then use the spray).

Pros:

- Great for securing hair in place.

- Will last the whole day.

- Won't make your hands stench with product residue.

Cons:

- Easy to overdo it and have your hair looking like it is made of cardboard.

- Difficult to remove as it needs plenty of water to soften back the hair.

- Not a good option for kinky hair (instead, use hair gel to harden the curls).

- You really don't want to get the stuff in your eyes (or your face, for that matter).

- Potential to inhale stuff you could do best without inhaling.

## Natural oils and butters

That's right, you can also use natural oils and butters to style your hair with! Coconut oil, olive oil, shea butter and jojoba oil are great agents to style your hair with, and they also aid in keeping your locks moisturised. Natural oils and butters provide the best results to those manes that are at least a medium length and are either coiled or kinky, although all hair types can benefit from natural oils and butter. Always use a minimal amount (think pea size) and approach using natural oils and butters to style your hair with a "less is more" attitude. Oils and butters can be used on any day of your hair-grooming schedule, and you can think of them as being natural complements to your own sebum. To use butters, simply melt your chosen one by rubbing your hands together (do not apply the butter in a solid state).

Pros:

- Will make your hair look slick and shiny.

- Will condition your hair as a natural complement to your sebum.

- Doesn't dry excessively.

- Will help in defining Ss, Es and Zs.

- Will add weight and thus help your hair hang down.

- Is a natural alternative, so you are ensured to not be absorbing unknown added chemicals through your scalp.

Cons:

- Extremely easy to overdo it and have your hair looking greasy.

- Not good for holding hair in place.

- Moderately difficult to remove (if you overdo it though, it will be a nightmare to remove).

- Takes longer to apply than other hairstyling agents as you have to be careful to not get the oil or butter on your scalp (same extra caution as with hair wax).

- Start with very small amounts for straight hair as it can make this hair type appear greasy very fast.

- Some natural oils and butters can give off a natural smell if you use too much (fancy walking around smelling like a coconut?).

- It can stain your shirt collars if you have medium or long-length hair and you use too much.

## How to style your hair

Ditch your hair brush, ditch it now!

To style your mane, you must use your fingers, a wide-tooth comb (for the curly hair types) or a conventional comb (straight hair). For most of the time, however, I recommend you to use your fingers solely and only rely on the wide-tooth/conventional comb for hairstyles in which you want your mane to be held in place (e.g. a swept or slicked hairstyle). Wide-tooth combs are also great for undoing hair tangles, so it is in your interest to own one if you have wavy, coiled or kinky hair; the best-quality wide-tooth combs are made out of wood or metal, avoid buying cheap plastic ones as they will chip easily.

With regards to applying your chosen hairstyling agent, coat your fingers with the agent and then run your fingers through your damp hair as you put your hair into your chosen hairstyle, trying to get most of the hairstyling agent on the segment of the hair strands from mid-shaft to the tip (as you'd do with conditioners). Once the hairstyling agent is applied and your hair has been styled with your fingers, you can then use the wide-tooth/conventional comb to give the finishing touches and directions to your mane, or you can continue using your fingers for the finishing touches of the hairstyle.

I must emphasise again that you have to use your chosen hairstyling agent on damp hair as this is a point that many men forget. Hairstyling agents won't work optimally on fully-dried hair, so having your mane damp is they way to go for its optimal styling with hairstyling agents. Once the hairstyling agent has been applied successfully to your damp hair, you are ready to leave the door with an awesome mane while your hair air-dries on its own to a fully-dried state as you go about your day.

## How to dry your hair after the shower

Part of the styling stage and a secondary action in itself, drying your hair is performed so as to take your hair from wet or soaked to damp. Typically, drying your hair occurs after you finish showering, and it is done prior to applying the hairstyling agents to your hair.

There are 2 options available to dry your hair: shaking your head or using a towel. The point of drying your hair is to remove the excess water from it so that you leave the hair damp; you should never dry your hair until it loses all the moisture gained from having wetted it in the first place.

The Shakeout is the colloquial name for shaking your head to remove the excess water and thus effectively dry your hair to a damp state without the use of a towel or cloth. As the name implies, you simply shake your head sideways and back and forth, allowing the water to drip from your hair. The Shakeout method is best used on medium and long-length hair since you need to have enough length to move the mass of hair as you shake your head. A spin-off of the Shakeout method is the Finger Shakeout: rapidly pass the fingers of both your hands over your hair, aiming to flick the water off the hair; the Finger Shakeout works best on short hair.

The second method is towel-drying, which is the preferred method for many males as it is more efficient than the Shakeout method in removing excess water. The main issue with towel-drying, however, is that it can cause tangling of your locks as well as frizz if not done right.

To optimally towel-dry, gently pass the towel over your mane as if you were literally caressing your scalp and hair, squeezing the hair with the towel in your hand to let the excess water drip. Do not vigorously rub the towel against your scalp because this will lead to the tangling of your mane and will make your hair frizz rapidly. It is very important that you gently pass the towel and squeeze your locks with the towel in your hand if you choose this hair-drying method. Moreover, I recommend you to use an old cotton T-shirt instead of a towel to dry your hair since most bath towels have a rough surface and cotton T-shirts are much smoother and easier on your hair (simply use cotton T-shirts that you no longer wear). Towel-drying is a great option for all hair lengths and hair types so long as you do it as recommended.

You can mix and match the hair-drying methods, but, whatever method you choose, the goal is to have your hair damp so as to be able to apply the hairstyling agent. After the hairstyling agent has been applied and the hair has been styled, you do not manipulate your hair further; the hair will slowly achieve a final look as it dries fully (i.e. air-dries) on its own over the course of a couple of hours. This is where the Damp vs. Dry (DvD) effect comes into play, and your hair will invariably look somewhat different once it has fully dried; it all depends on your hair type, hair length, chosen hairstyle, chosen hairstyling agent, and your unique Curl Factor.

## A note on using hair dryers

You are probably aware of what a hair dryer is, if anything because any of the females in your life (sister, mother or girlfriend/wife) quite likely has one and uses it frequently. Hair dryers, also known as blow dryers, are tools used to further dry your hair rapidly when your hair is damp instead of having to wait the few hours that your locks may take to fully air-dry on their own. Hair dryers are also of use for enhancing the volume of your hair and putting your mane into elaborate hairstyles.

The main problem with hair dryers is that these artefacts rely on the blowing of hot air to work their fast-drying magic. Excessive heat, especially as given out by hair dryers, can damage your hair over the long term particularly if your hair care is subpar. If you want to use a hair dryer to dry your hair or enhance a hairstyle, follow these points:

- Use the coldest temperature available in the settings.

- Clip a diffuser to the hair drier to allow for optimal dissipation of the air expelled.

- Coat your hair with a special heat-protecting hair product prior to using the hair dryer.

- Do not use the hair dryer on wet or soaked hair; always dry your hair to a damp state (via the Shakeout or towel-drying) prior to drying your hair with the hair dryer.

- Do not go all out with the hair dryer to completely dry your hair, leave some moisture (i.e. dampness) in the hair as otherwise your hair will end up resembling a dead rat!

I recommend you to leave hair dryers out of the daily hair-grooming equation and instead use these tools for specific occasions (e.g. when you want to rock a certain hairstyle). Hair dryers will do more bad than good if used daily as such frequent use will irreversibly damage your hair. For your daily hair grooming, use any of the 2 aforementioned hair-drying methods (Shakeout and/or towel-drying), and allow your mane to fully air-dry naturally as you go about your day.

## The 9-Minute Perfect Mane routine

To approach the grooming of your hair, you must regard the process as a routine. This is because grooming your locks is inherently a daily sequence of main and secondary actions, and, to become better at something, you need to practise it frequently and in an orderly fashion; there's no 2 ways about this. What's more is that your hair-grooming routine will vary in a slightly different manner according to the day as you alter the secondary actions in the 3 hair-grooming stages. Regardless, your hair-grooming routine will be built upon the template of having the 3 stages and main actions of cleaning, conditioning and styling performed on a daily basis. If you need another quick visual reference, see the table on Figure 19 (in the beginning of the chapter) for the 3 stages and their secondary actions (it is also found as Appendix XIX in the Appendix).

Of course, throughout the years, I have perfected my own hair-grooming routine. Because I like to be my own lab rat and because all the hair-grooming advice out there for guys involves massive amounts of time investment, I decided to really work on a hair-grooming routine that would be convenient and that would yield great cosmetic results. This hair-grooming routine that I came up with and perfected is called the 9-Minute Perfect Mane routine, and it involves everything you have read in this hair-grooming chapter, albeit put together in a convenient and methodical manner. The 9-Minute Perfect Mane routine acts as the initial template to use for your hair-management efforts since it comprises the 3 hair-grooming stages and helps you to visualise the flow of secondary actions.

I have been able to use the 9-Minute Perfect Mane routine while living in different countries, working on my career, training for a sport and partying my derriere off, so, with this hair-grooming routine, you have the 3 hair-grooming stages assembled into a convenient and optimal order and flow, ultimately suiting modern males like you and I who need time efficiency slammed into their daily hair management. The 9-Minute Perfect Mane routine is ideally done in a bathroom setting as it integrates the whole hair-grooming process and shampooing is best done in the shower.

Here is the 9-Minute Perfect Mane routine, step by step (TT means Time Taken):

1.    Jump in the shower. For best results, water should be lukewarm. Singing is recommended to get into the routine. (TT: 10 seconds)

2.    Soak your hair with running water. Hair must be soaked in its entirety. (TT: 30 seconds)

3.    Grab the shampoo. Squeeze out a fingertip amount and place it on the centre of the top of your head. (TT: 10 seconds)

4.    Repeat Step 3 on your other 5 scalp segments: both sides of head, front, vertex and the area 4 inches above the nape. (TT: 50 seconds)

5.    Pair the segments of the scalp and massage each segment with each hand simultaneously. Spread the shampoo to a 4-inch radius as you massage in a circular motion. Each paired segment is massaged for a count of 20 seconds. (TT: 60 seconds)

6.    Rinse the shampoo with your head tilted forward or backward. (TT: 30 seconds)

7.    Possibly change the song you've been singing. Up to you, but do it immediately.

8.    Grab the normal conditioner and squeeze it out on your fingers so that they (fingers) are coated in a thick film of conditioner. (TT: 10 seconds)

9.    Work your fingers through your locks from mid-length to the tip, coating the hair plentifully with conditioner. (TT: 60 seconds)

10.    Now clean your body. Make sure that you take 2 minutes to clean your body, which is the time that the conditioner should be left on your hair without rinsing. (TT: 120 seconds)

11.    Rinse the conditioner. (TT: 30 seconds)

12.    Get out of the shower. You are now going to style that mane. Start singing a new song if you so desire. (TT: 20 seconds)

13.    Dry your hair via the Shakeout method and/or with a towel or cotton T-shirt so that your mane is left damp. (TT: 30 seconds)

14.    Grab your chosen hairstyling agent and put some on your fingers. (TT: 10 seconds)

15.    Run your fingers through your locks and style your mane as desired. Make sure that you don't get any of the hairstyling agent on the scalp. (TT: 60 seconds)

16.    Wink at yourself. You are looking great and are ready to take the day with that awesome mane of yours.

The 9-Minute Perfect Mane routine contains 16 fluid steps and takes 530 seconds or 10 seconds under 9 minutes, from the moment you are about to get in the shower to the moment your hair is set and ready to go. Oh, and that is only on the days that you use shampoo; on your non-shampooing days, your average 9-Minute Perfect Mane routine can take even less (see Appendix XXV for reference). The above 9-Minute Perfect Mane routine serves as your initial template to then start modifying the secondary hair-grooming actions to fit the routine according to your mane's needs and preferences as well as whether it is a shampooing or non-shampooing day.

The 9-Minute Perfect Mane routine has you, in less than 9 minutes, sporting great-looking hair so that you can then get on with the rest of your day. We are talking less than 9 minutes to have a head of locks that looks awesome, a mane that you will be proud to be leaving the house with. Even with my own bushy coils and kinks, I still manage it in less than 9 minutes. If I can do it with this beast, you too can do it, and, as you master the 9-Minute Perfect Mane routine, you will be able to gradually trim your routine's time to mere minutes.

In the beginning, the 9-Minute Perfect Mane routine will take you more than 9 minutes, and that is absolutely normal. With practice comes perfect, and your goal is to get better at grooming your mane in all of the 3 stages comprising your hair-grooming routine. Give yourself plenty of time to get your hair grooming down to 9 minutes or less. Stay focused and aim to drop your hair-grooming time slowly by following the 9-Minute Perfect Mane routine's template; eventually you will get to the 9-minute mark, all you need is some hands-on experience.

Most men complain about the time that it takes them to tame their hair, yet the problem is not their hair itself, the problem is the way in which they approach their daily hair grooming. The way that I am showing you to approach your hair grooming is the tried and tested method to live in our modern day with a mane of locks that is both aesthetic and convenient. We all want convenience without sacrificing cosmetic results, and, with the 9-Minute Perfect Mane routine, you will get the best of both worlds.

To illustrate how much you will benefit from this routine, I know ladies who spend 60 minutes on their hair before leaving the bathroom because the expert whom they read claims that doing so will give them superbly-defined fabulous curls. I also know plenty of men who just buzz their hair to a #1 every 2 weeks because they claim that it is impossible to manage their hair without spending a considerable amount of their morning managing their heads. Baloney, I say!

With the 9-Minute Perfect Mane routine and all the knowledge you have garnered so far, you will be able to get those locks looking the part while being able to devote all the time that you saved to either getting on time to work or doing manly stuff like hitting the gym hard and doing extracurricular bedroom activities. That's how I use my saved time, and that is how you should use it too!

# Wrapping up your hair-grooming routine

The 9-Minute Perfect Mane routine is a template that outlines the optimal order in which to base your cleaning, conditioning and styling stages. As laid out in the template, the 9-Minute Perfect Mane routine illustrates a typical shampooing day: you shampoo, then you condition, and then you move to styling your hair. Typically, your shampooing days will be longer than your non-shampooing days although the 9-Minute Perfect Mane routine is fully customisable according to your own needs and preferences, so you can make it last pretty much as long as you want.

Your hair-grooming routine is always consistent in its sequence, goals, and emphasis on the 3 hair-grooming main actions, but it will differ somewhat according to the day of the week as you remove or add secondary actions on each day; indeed, this adding and removing of secondary actions in your routine will depend, among other variables, on your shampooing frequency, conditioning frequency, a greater need for the Sebum Coating method or whether you want to style your hair or go solo (i.e. no hairstyling agent).

By now, you are ready to start creating your own hair-grooming routine using the template for the 9-Minute Perfect Mane routine, adding or removing secondary actions on each day as you see fit, but, at all times, maintaining an emphasis on the main actions of cleaning, conditioning and styling.

For example, the Sebum Coating method has not been mentioned in the template for the 9-Minute Perfect Mane routine, but you know from reading this chapter that the Sebum Coating method is performed on your non-shampooing days, that the Sebum Coating method precedes the conditioning stage, that the Sebum Coating method has an inherent cleaning and conditioning action, and that the Sebum Coating method is the first secondary action that you implement on non-shampooing days. Furthermore, you can remove the conditioning stage on your non-shampooing days and be left with just the Sebum Coating method and the styling stage; you can even skip using any hairstyling agents for your mane and just do the Sebum Coating method, dry your hair and go hairstyle free on your non-shampooing days; it's that customisable!

I have attached in the Appendix (Appendix XXV) a table that illustrates what a hair-grooming routine based on a 1 on/1 off shampooing frequency can look like when put into a week. It illustrates how each day has its own 9-Minute Perfect Mane routine albeit with variations in secondary actions while maintaining the focus on cleaning, conditioning and styling. The table also allows you to visualise the importance of having a hair-grooming routine as you can see how each day of the week follows on to the next by taking into account what has been implemented the day before and what is to be implemented the day after.

The best way to create your hair-grooming routine is to do so by building it around your shampooing frequency and using the template of the 9-Minute Perfect Mane routine on your shampooing days. Leave the conditioning frequency without experimenting until you find out your optimal shampooing frequency, and follow the initial guideline of only using a normal conditioner after the rinsing of the shampoo (i.e. on your shampooing days), then proceeding with the styling stage. Once you have sorted out your shampooing frequency, then you can start introducing the normal conditioner on your non-shampooing days as you desire.

On your non-shampooing days, start by using the Sebum Coating method, which does the cleaning and conditioning actions, then moving to the styling stage to be implemented with a leave-in conditioner and your chosen hairstyling agent. As it goes, the conditioning action on your non-shampooing days is provided by both the Sebum Coating method and the leave-in conditioner; the 3 stages and their main actions are satisfied because the Sebum Coating does the cleaning and conditioning while the leave-in also does the conditioning and provides the styling. What counts is that the sequence of the 3 main actions is respected so as to have an optimal hair-grooming routine, whether it is a shampooing or non-shampooing day.

Going by the above, you can now see the importance of striving to find out your optimal shampooing frequency as your hair-grooming routine is based around this hair-cleaning element. As you take the time to find out your optimal shampooing frequency, use the sequences of secondary actions for your shampooing and non-shampooing days that are illustrated in Figure 21, and, once you have found out your optimal shampooing frequency, it is then that you can start customising the secondary actions to your desire such as increasing the frequency of use of normal and leave-in conditioners, using more hairstyling agents or inserting the Sebum Coating method on more days.

Figure 21 – Generic guidelines to start your hair-grooming routine

| STAGES | SHAMPOOING DAY | NON-SHAMPOOING DAY |
|---|---|---|
| *Cleaning* | Shampoo | Sebum Coating method (dual action) |
| *Conditioning* | Normal conditioner | |
| *Styling* | Yes | Yes |
| *Leave-in conditioner?* | No (style with other hairstyling agent) | Yes (style with leave-in + other hairstyling agent) |

Overall, when you start customising your hair-grooming routine, stick to the initial guidelines of Figure 21 above for your shampooing and non-shampooing days and don't do any experiments with your secondary actions until you have secured your optimal shampooing frequency. Once secured, you can modify your routine but always abiding by the sequence of the hair-grooming process and using a "trial and error" mindset in that if you experience regression of results, you must react promptly and undo any changes that have caused the regression.

Lastly, the same 3 tables in the Appendix (Appendix XXVII, Appendix XXVIII and Appendix XIX) that I referenced at the beginning of this section have all the key elements of your hair-grooming routine so that you can use a visual reference as you learn and apply all the content in this chapter. The tables are specific to the hair-length categories and provide guidelines for everything concerning your hair-grooming routine. It is now that you have finished this chapter that you can study these tables and understand them; thus, these tables are of special relevance when first setting up your hair-grooming routine although any time that you modify your routine and find yourself having doubts, you can go back to the hair-grooming guidelines in the tables as a new starting point.

## **Conclusion**

Your hair-grooming aspect needs to be regarded as a daily process. You must ensure that you do the stipulated 3 stages every day, and you must choose your secondary actions accordingly.

Altogether, your hair-grooming schedule will be dependent upon your shampooing frequency, which is the most crucial element of all of your hair grooming. Aim to find out your shampooing frequency while using the aforementioned generic hair-grooming schedule; once you find out your shampooing frequency, then start playing around with the secondary actions.

For your styling, it is more important that you know what hairstyling agents you have available and how to style your hair than actually knowing specific hairstyles. However, you will find the range of hairstyles available for your hair type in Chapter 6.

It is once you get your hair-grooming elements honed that you will be able to put your hair grooming on auto-pilot. Literally, you will be taking mere minutes every day to have your hair looking how you want it to look!

## Anthony's barbershop case study

Jael was a male in his teens who had kinky hair and was tired of getting his usual buzz cuts. He had come to Anthony looking to improve his hair; he wanted an alternative to the same boring buzz cuts he had been getting every 2 weeks for years. Jael's main problem was that he didn't know how to groom his hair every day hence the buzz cuts.

In order to give Jael the best advice, Anthony had Jael first know about his hair type and had Jael understand that he needs to be realistic about what can be done and what can't be done with his hair. The way Anthony saw it was that it would only be once Jael knew how to manage his hair daily that he (Jael) would be able to start looking into suitable hairstyles for his kinks.

Jael's case was typical: a male who had curly hair and had tried to grow his hair a bit, only to find that it was impossible to have his hair looking somewhat aesthetic. The first action Anthony recommended was for Jael to find out his optimal shampooing frequency, a hair-grooming element that is ignored by the vast majority of curly-haired males. Thus, Jael went on an 8-weeks-long mission to optimally find his shampooing frequency, visiting Anthony every 2 weeks to keep his kinks at the same length. Jael found out that, as a kinky-haired male, he needed a frequency of 1 on/7 off to have his mane most moisturised; his chosen hairstyling agent during this period of time was coconut butter in tiny amounts to coat the tips of his curls, and he found out that coconut butter plus a leave-in conditioner was the perfect blend of hairstyling agents for his kinky hair.

Some months later, Jael was able to grow a cool, lengthy Afro (6 inches long) that had women asking him about his hair grooming all the time!

# 4) Hair-Care Aspect: The Big 3 Issues To Battle To Sport Great-Looking Hair

In this chapter, I will cover how to keep your hair looking healthy and in optimal condition over the long term. While knowing your hair grooming and having a hair-grooming routine is a must to get those locks looking awesome, you also need to address the optimal hair care of your mane in the long run, meaning that you must know the ins and outs of dealing 24/7 with a great-looking head of hair. Essentially, hair grooming yields instant cosmetic results while hair care yields cumulative cosmetic benefits and optimises the health aspect of your mane. Hair grooming and hair care go together in ultimately achieving great-looking hair, but it is important to have them separated and have a chapter dedicated to each so that you can see them as different key aspects of your goal of great hair.

Having said all of the above, the use of the word "health" in this chapter is not literal. By "hair health", I will be referring to how your hair keeps its good looks in the long run, and the healthy and vigorous impression that it will exude. Have you ever taken a look at whatever cover dude is on the latest men's magazine and thought how his hair looked uber healthy? Apart from all the Photoshop retouching, it is not that his hair strands breathe in glorious amounts of oxygen or that his hair shafts are coated in nutritional blends engineered in some obscure laboratory. Nope, not even close; the dude just happens to know how to take care of his hair (that, or his image and PR teams know how to take care of his hair), thus his mane gets to look healthy.

Your hair can be made to look better, smoother and glossier (and thus, look "healthy") by not only grooming it properly but also by taking care of it when you go about your day-to-day business. Moreover, since hair doesn't have an ability to repair itself (as opposed to how skin does), the trick is to avoid damaging the hair in the first place, thus your hair care must have an special emphasis on preventing rather than fixing and should be seen as a strategy, for it will include a set of measures to be implemented long term.

With hair care, there is also a nutritional component that is of the utmost relevance and that is most commonly left out when men think of ways to look after their hair.

Since the real living part of your hair is the follicle, the best hair-care tactic to use so as to grow stronger and healthier-looking hair strands is to feed the follicle optimally, and this is done via your nutritional approach: the sum of the foods you eat plus the nutritional supplements you may take. Altogether, the nutrients that you provide your body with via your nutritional approach nourish the tiny hair-producing factories that each hair follicle is. Considering that there are more than 100,000 follicles in the average male head, you've got some nourishing to do!

This chapter specifically deals with the issues that you will be encountering with your hair over the long term, and I will cover all the hair-care measures available to you so as to ensure that these issues do not impact the looks and health of your mane. The next chapter will look at your nutrition, which is an essential part of your hair care, and you will learn all about the diet and the nutritional supplementation that has worked for me to make the most of my locks. Altogether, your hair-care measures and your nutrition make up your hair-care strategy and hair-care aspect, for which its optimisation will be your ticket to a long-lasting mane.

## The Big 3 mane issues

As part of sporting great-looking hair, your daily hair care will be centred around preventing and addressing the following 3 issues:

1.  Dry hair

2.  Tangled hair

3.  Hair loss (specifically, male pattern baldness)

You will encounter the issue of dry hair on a daily basis while tangled hair will be more notorious if you have any of the curly hair types (wavy, coiled or kinky). The third issue is included because hair loss is a serious issue that most men will experience sooner or later and that can be managed from the first day, even if you are not currently suffering from it.

Alone or in combination, these 3 issues have the potential to ruin the most optimally-groomed of all heads of hair, yet you must not be put off by these bad boys as they are issues that all males will experience, whether they already have great-looking hair, a dead rat or simply want to tame the beast with a buzz cut. The good news is that a good hair-care strategy will battle and minimise these issues while helping immensely in taking your mane to the epic level that it should be at.

To fight these 3 issues on a daily basis, you have to think of hair-care measures, and I have put these measures into 2 categories: proactive and reactive. Proactive measures imply actions that are taken to avoid issues happening in the first place while reactive measures imply actions that are taken to directly address the issue when it has happened. Proactive measures tend to be associated with the hair-grooming process whereas reactive measures are part of a more ad hoc approach, for you will be performing your reactive measures to fix a problem instead of purposely preventing it as with proactive measures.

The emphasis placed on these proactive and reactive measures will become more important as you grow your mane into the medium and long lengths. Near-shaved and short-length hair can get away with skipping some of the hair-care measures or not being as careful, but I highly recommend you to follow all described measures regardless of your hair length or hair type if you want to ensure the never-ending optimal health of your head of luscious locks.

As men desiring greatness when it comes to our hair, it isn't just what we do in the bathroom that matters. Once we step outside, we must also keep an eye on our manes because the elements are always working against our optimised hair. Through my years of experimenting, banging my head against the wall and shaving my head only to grow my locks again, I have been able to come up with these proactive and reactive hair-care measures specific to each of the Big 3 mane issues.

## Dry hair

Battling this bad boy is your main goal when it comes to hair care. Dry hair is easy to identify as it feels like hay, is frizzy and brittle, and the shape of the locks is not defined. The opposite of dry hair is moisturised hair: your Is, Ss, Es or Zs will feel light and smooth, look more defined and will be much easier to manage. Do not confuse, however, dry hair with drying your hair: the latter is part of your hair-grooming routine and aims to remove excess water from the hair so as to leave it damp (thus, with moisturise), whereas the former (dry hair) is hair that has been stripped of moisture and is the result of improper hair care and a subpar hair-grooming routine.

I always say this, if you can keep your hair from losing its moisture and becoming dry in the first place, you will have solved 99% of your hair-related worries. While all hair types have the potential to become dry and be plagued with dryness and lack of moisture, the degree of predisposition to becoming dry ranges between hair types. The predisposition range is as follow (least predisposed first, most predisposed last):

1. Straight hair (least predisposed)

2. Wavy hair

3. Coiled hair

4. Kinky hair (most predisposed)

As you can see, the more naturally-curving the hair type is, the higher its propensity to become dry will be, hence the reason for so many curly-haired males walking around with frizzy hair. Dry hair is brittle and frizzy, and the locks will interlock (i.e. tangle and knot) easily, which is exactly the opposite of what we want.

Luckily for us, there are hair-care measures, both proactive and reactive, that will put an end to dry hair. Dry hair takes days to manifest if it is occurring from an already-moisturised mane, so you will be able to notice daily in the mirror how your hair slowly becomes dry, thus allowing you to tackle this issue before it gets really bad.

Proactive:

• Go easy on very hot environments. This means saunas, very hot showers or extreme temperatures (think desert type). As a modern male, it is impossible to avoid these environments unless you want to live a life of boredom so just don't go crazy on them, especially saunas (e.g. don't hit the sauna for extended periods of time on a daily basis).

• Stop shampooing every day. Drop your shampooing frequency; really aim to find your optimal frequency as described in the previous hair-grooming chapter. This measure works rapidly and extremely well to prevent the risk of your hair becoming dry.

- Use a leave-in conditioner for much of your hair-grooming efforts. Try to change your hairstyles to those that are optimally styled with a leave-in alone or in conjunction with other hairstyling agents (apply the leave-in conditioner first). Hairstyles that are favoured by leave-in conditioners are those where the hair doesn't have to be held in a gravity-defying position.

- Do not blow-dry your hair on a daily basis. If you want to use a hair dryer (i.e. blow-dry your hair), clip a diffuser to it, coat your hair priorly with a heat-protecting hair product and use the coldest temperature available in the settings. Furthermore, never blow-dry wet or soaked hair, only blow-dry your hair when it is damp.

- Use a normal conditioner after shampooing, and, once you have your optimal shampooing frequency worked out, play with increasing your conditioning frequency. Normal conditioners only take 2 minutes to be left on as you continue to shower, and, if you master the 9-Minute Perfect mane routine, your busiest hair-grooming day will take less than 9 minutes.

- Aim to wet your hair every day, regardless of whether it is a shampooing or non-shampooing day. Water plus your sebum and/or an artificial conditioner equates moisturised hair strands.

- Do not alter your hair: don't straighten it, bleach it or do anything to permanently alter its texture or structure. Altering your hair will damage it, weaken it and make it more prone to dryness. It will also destroy your natural curl pattern if you have wavy, coiled or kinky hair, making it harder to have defined curls.

Reactive:

- If you currently have hair that has been straightened permanently, or if you have been using hair-straightening gadgets (e.g. flat irons), it is a good idea to start from a fresh batch of hair. Cut your hair and start growing new hair that will now be managed optimally.

- When you find your hair starting to look dry, schedule a normal-conditioner session (i.e. the secondary action of using a normal conditioner) as soon as possible. It can be on the same day or a few days later, just don't delay it for more than 3 days.

- Shampoo before the scheduled conditioner session, then don't shampoo again for the next 7 days. After the stipulated 7-day period of no shampooing, go back to your usual shampooing frequency.

- For the next 7 days after you initially address your dry hair, use a normal conditioner on every day and hit the leave-in conditioner extra hard on all 7 days (i.e. use it every day and in copious amounts).

- Make sure to also do the Sebum Coating method every day for these 7 days (remember, the Sebum Coating method is always the first secondary action you do on any day).

- If you are starting your awesome-mane journey with very dry hair, I advise you to use a deep conditioner every 2 weeks for the next 8 weeks. Deep conditioners are stronger forms of normal conditioners, and you will find them next to normal conditioners in wherever it is that you buy your hair products from. You can also use a hair mask instead of a deep conditioner if you so prefer.

## Tangled hair

Your hair will tangle and form knots, that's a reality. Together with dry hair, the sooner you accept and face this fact, the sooner you will get your hair care going. Just like with dry hair, tangled hair is best managed with proactive measures because improperly-cared hair can tangle very bad, to the point that the tangled mess has to be chopped. Tangles tend to precede knots; that is, your hair will first tangle and, if left unaddressed, the tangle will morph into knots, with this metamorphosis being most notorious in coiled and kinky hair.

Tangled hair can actually form hair knots that are, to put it bluntly, evil. I have experienced some cunningly formed knots over the years that I had to ultimately chop as I perfected my proactive measures although nowadays I got so good at it that I seldom get an evil tangled lock (I normally get them when I do experiments). For the record, chopping a tangle or hair knot should always be the last resort, always!

Incidentally, having dry hair will further magnify your risk of tangling. Thus, keeping your mane moisturised and dry free is in itself a great proactive measure, but it will not totally protect you from developing some nasty tangles, hence you need to emphasise your tangled-hair proactive measures at all costs. Moreover, an excess build up of sebum or hairstyling agents can cause your hair to tangle too, thus the importance of finding out and having an optimal shampooing frequency.

Your hair will also have the tendency to tangle more the longer it is. Expect to have to put yourself to use with this "tangling" matter on a frequent basis once your mane hits a long length. If you want to grow your hair to a long length and beyond, be prepared to find a few tangles every day despite your proactive efforts. That's the nature of the long-haired beast!

Once you find a tangled or knotted lock of hair, you must approach the detangling task like a surgeon would approach an operation, which is why I truly want you to see cutting the tangled hair as a last measure: a good surgeon never gives up on his patient! Detangling is in itself an art, and the more you practise it, the better you will get at it, just like with hair grooming.

Detangling requires you to softly pull the length of the hair that precedes the tangle or knot and use a pulling motion that goes towards the direction of the scalp. You must use plenty of conditioner or natural oils to grease the tangle priorly, which means that detangling is just an awful and messy procedure altogether and is best avoided. Thus, you must do all within reach to work your proactive measures hard. Be aware that some of the following measures are a bit annoying, and it is up to you whether you want to apply them or not; ultimately, the more you use them, the better your mane will look.

Proactive:

- Run your fingers through your hair strands every time that you use a normal conditioner. Apply the conditioner to your hair, and run your fingers or wide-tooth comb from the scalp down the tips. You can do this measure as you see fit, for you can do it during the 2 minutes that the normal conditioner has to be left on the hair (conditioning stage) and you can also do it when you are applying the leave-in conditioner (styling stage). Unlike in the Sebum Coating method where your fingers are placed in a pinching manner, you detangle your hair with your fingers forming a rake, which essentially mimics a wide-tooth comb. Thus, either use your fingers or a wide-tooth comb for this proactive measure.

- Tie your hair when you go to bed. This is only applicable to those with medium or long-length hair. Secure your locks into a ponytail or, better yet, into a bun or braid. Use a hair band, do not use any rubber band you find around. If the length of your mane is not enough to tie all of the hair into one bun, then don't be afraid to tie your hair into 2, 3 or even 4 buns. Just warn anyone who may see you the next morning when you wake up (you can skip this measure for one-night stands!).

- If your hair is of a short length, then you can use a dorag or sleeping hair cap to secure your mane and avoid the hair being loose. While sleeping caps are traditionally associated with women and weird hair potions, sleeping caps are secretly used by quite a good portion of men who know of the sleeping cap's benefits in avoiding tangled hair. I have used them in the past though for the most part I prefer to go solo (i.e. no hair cap) if my hair is short.

- For bedtime, I also recommend you to sleep on pillow cases made of satin or silk. The former is not very expensive and will help prevent your mane from tangling at night. Silk is very comfortable and smooth to have your head resting on but is obviously the more expensive option. These 2 types of fabric reduce the friction on your hair from rubbing your head on the pillow as you sleep, which aids greatly in discouraging the tangling of your locks.

- Use a leave-in conditioner most of the time for your styling. Not only is this hairstyling agent great for adding extra conditioning to your locks but it is also great for adding extra slip to your hair and avoiding the risk of tangling. Apply the leave-in first and then apply your other chosen hairstyling agents.

- When drying your mane, avoid using a conventional towel. Use a 100% cotton T-shirt instead, and you can do like me and buy a few cheap ones, which you'll use solely for drying your hair. If you use a conventional towel, do as I recommend in the previous chapter and smoothly pass the towel over your locks as you squeeze them; never rub the towel vigorously against your hair as this is a sure way to get your hair frizzy and tangled in an instant! There are also some bath towels that don't have rough surfaces, and you can use this type of towels if you'd rather dry your hair with a towel than with a T-shirt.

- Tie your mane on windy days. If you cannot tie your hair, use plenty of leave-in conditioner before you leave the house. Same goes for driving a convertible car, tie your hair or use a leave-in conditioner. I still remember when I took a date out in my convertible some years ago while I was still learning about my hair: I started the date with my mane looking great, and, by the end of the drive, I was sporting a full-on dead rat atop my head. Lesson learnt, tie your hair or use a leave-in conditioner if you are going to be in a windy environment.

- Avoid unnecessarily rubbing your head against surfaces such as head rests or couches. This one is a bit excessive, and, if you can't be bothered to use this measure, at least tie your hair if you have medium/long-length hair. For example, I would tie my medium-length curls every time that I would go for long car rides.

- Once your hair gets to hang down, try to keep it tied for a good portion of your day. The more the hair is hanging down and dangling, the more the chances of tangling.

Reactive:

- Tackle a tangle/knot as soon as you spot it. The longer you wait, the worse it will get.

- Before detangling, use either a normal conditioner or a natural oil to coat the tangle and provide slip. Don't only coat the tangle, coat the whole lock of hair in which the tangle is found. Coconut oil and olive oil work great as natural oils to provide slip.

- When detangling, pull softly the tangled hair towards the scalp with one hand as you pinch the tangle/knot firmly with the other hand. It is preferable that you use your fingers for this measure instead of a wide-tooth comb; the wide-tooth comb is best used as a rake for your proactive measures.

- If the tangle is big and you find it hard to detangle, pour apple-cider vinegar on the tangle and leave the vinegar on the tangle without rinsing for 5 minutes. One of the reasons for tangles to form is due to an overaccumulation of sebum that has hardened; the apple-cider vinegar works to soften the sebum, allowing for better detangling. After the stipulated 5 minutes, rinse the vinegar, and then coat the tangle with normal conditioner or oil to continue detangling.

- Chopping is the last option; even very bad tangles can be fixed with patience, and you can work them in separate sessions instead of in a single session. You may find at times, however, a tangle so viciously formed that you will just have to chop it off. Weigh the pros and cons of doing this and remember that the tangled hair will continue to tangle more and more if you don't do anything about it immediately. Sometimes, you will just have to give up on your follicular patient!

- Once you have detangled the lock, wet it and coat it with normal conditioner. If you had to work through several tangles in that session, soak all of your hair in water and apply normal conditioner to all of your mane. Rinse the conditioner as usual after 2 minutes, then apply a leave-in conditioner to the hair. Resume your hair-grooming schedule the next day.

## Hair loss

This one is a big issue for us men, and there are 2 main forms of hair loss that you will be facing with your straight, wavy, coiled or kinky-haired mane: shedding and balding.

110

Shedding is a natural scalp process in which a given hair strand detaches itself from the scalp while the rest of hair strands in the scalp continue to grow. Shedding is part of a healthy follicle's life cycle, and each hair strand in your scalp has an expiration date; at the end of the hair's life cycle, the hair strand simply detaches itself, making room in the follicle for a new hair strand to grow from scratch. On average, males shed about 100 hair strands per day, and you will notice a lot of shed hairs in the shower or everywhere in the house once you start taking good care of your hair.

When one doesn't groom his hair properly, one carries around plenty of shed hairs that are, in fact, trapped in the remaining growing hair strands that make one's mane. What all of this means is that, in an improperly-groomed head of Is, Ss, Es or Zs, most shed hairs have yet to fall off despite being effectively detached from the hair follicles. It is once you start using conditioners and keeping your locks optimally coated with sebum that you will start seeing more hairs falling off than usual. Do not worry; increased apparent shedding when you first start to use conditioners optimally is completely normal as your moisturised locks will now have more slip and the shed hairs will be allowed to fall off instead of remaining trapped in your mane. The visibility of your shed hairs will also be exacerbated if you grow your hair to a medium or long length (the longer your hair is, the more visible the shed hairs will be).

The other relevant form of hair loss is balding: a hair loss process that is not part of the healthy life cycle of a hair strand (as opposed to hair shedding) and that can be caused by several factors including one's genes, certain medications, stress, disease or hormones. To us men, the most important form of balding is male pattern baldness (MPB); the form of permanent balding that men experience due to being, well, men!

As you have learnt in Chapter 2 "Hair-Profiling Aspect: Get To Know Your Hair!", your body as a male produces several sex hormones, and one of them, dihydrotestosterone (DHT), is one of the culprits behind MPB. Dihydrotestosterone is responsible for giving you your masculine attributes (e.g. a deep voice or thick hair covering your body), but it also has the negative effect of slowly killing away your hair follicles. The MPB process is not fully understood, but research points to DHT and inherited genes being two of the key pieces in the MPB puzzle. For what is worth, your own unique genetic response to DHT is what will ultimately predispose you to MPB; just because you have high levels of DHT, it doesn't mean that you will go bald.

Male pattern baldness is a slow process that is actually classified in stages so as to gauge its evolution. In Chapter 2, I introduced to you the Hamilton-Norwood scale pioneered by Dr. James Hamilton in the '50s, and later revised by Dr. O'Tar Norwood in the '70s. Also simplified and known as the Norwood scale, this staging method classifies MPB in 7 progressive stages starting with recession of the forehead's hairline towards the vertex and increased frontal hair thinning (Stage I to II), and finishing with no hair at all on the top and back of the head (Stage VII). Since MPB will commonly begin at both sides of the forehead's hairline (i.e. the temples), it is easy for MPB to go unnoticed in its initial stages; this being the reason behind my emphasis on keeping a close eye on one's hairline if MPB runs in the family. I recommend you to fully research the topic of male pattern baldness as there are some good online and offline resources to learn from, and it is imperative for you to see a good dermatologist or medical specialist if you suspect MPB.

For our third issue of hair loss, I will give you the proactive and reactive measures to primarily guard yourself against MPB although you will also find some lifestyle choices that will help towards preventing not only MPB but also hair loss attributed to stress and other external factors. With regards to hair shedding, you have nothing to worry about as, again, it is a completely natural process.

Proactive:

- If MPB runs in your family and you are over the age of 18, start taking photos of your hairline. Take pictures every 3 months of the front, top, side and back of your head. If MPB doesn't run in your family, yet you are concerned about losing your hair, take pictures every 6 months instead. Compare the pictures that you have taken over time: any receding at the temples and lowered hair density that is noticed is a sign of MPB.

- Since MPB has a strong inherited component, do some family investigation and try to speak to family members to know which males in the family line have gone bald and at what age (go back a few generations). Contrary to popular belief, MPB can be passed from both the maternal and the paternal lineage, not just the mother's side as the myth goes. Also, if any males in the last 2 generations of your family tree have gone bald before the age of 35, it will mean that there is a strong MPB predisposition in the family so keep a close eye

*(follows from previous page)*

on your hair as advised in the previous point.

- Read as much as you can on MPB. Be aware, however, that the hair-loss industry is full of scammers and snake-oil products. Keep an eye on my sites among other sources for trusted content on MPB.

- If you tie your hair, make sure to not tie it tight. When you tie your hair, release tension from the follicles by slightly and smoothly pulling the tied hair against the direction of the ponytail/bun/braid. You can actually lose hair from leaving your hair tied too tight, with this particular form of hair loss being known as traction alopecia.

- If you have wavy, coiled or kinky hair, avoid hair brushes and conventional/pocket combs. Only use your fingers or a wide-tooth comb to style your curls. Hair brushes and conventional/pocket combs will have you pulling your curls excessively, which will damage the hair strands and follicles.

- If your hair shedding is getting out of hand, start keeping a close eye on your hairline as well as on the hair density on top of your head. Intense emotional stress or distraught can bring about a temporary increase in hair shedding, and the hair loss will not follow the predictable temple recession of MPB. In any case, monitor your hairline and hair density as MPB is the form of hair loss that is most relevant to you, for it is irreversible.

- Avoid hairstyles that have you pulling your hair too hard, such as excessively side parting your locks so that your hair looks flat. Again, avoid any excessive pulling of your hair and choose hairstyles that do not require you to manipulate your hair too much especially if you already suffer from MPB.

- Make sure that your diet is spot on. This means eating a healthy diet emphasising a good amount of protein and fish oils as well as an optimal intake of micronutrients (i.e. minerals and vitamins). An optimal diet will not only ensure that your hair grows its strongest and healthiest but will also ensure that you add years to your mane's lifetime; likewise, there are several nutritional supplements that can be used to bulletproof your diet and maximise

*(follows from previous page)*

the nourishment of your hair from within. The next chapter covers all about your optimal diet and supplement use for your mane.

- Exercise improves blood circulation, and one of the theories explaining MPB goes that this form of hair loss is partially caused by an inadequate supply of blood flow to the hair follicles. While it would be a wild exaggeration to directly link exercising with the curing of MPB, it will not do you any damage to exercise frequently so that you pair a great-looking mane with a great-looking and healthy body. If exercising does provide a benefit to male pattern baldness (however small the benefit may be), then you'll at least have killed 2 birds with 1 stone!

- I know it sounds easier said than done but try to minimise high levels of chronic stress. Chronic stress not only exacerbates hair loss but it also makes you age faster and decreases your quality of life. Ask yourself, does this added stress bring a benefit to any area of my life? Life is about balance, harmony and taking actions, so carefully analyse and evaluate the pros and cons of living your life with high levels of stress.

- Research your medications. There are many medications that list hair loss as a side effect and concomitant use of medications that can cause hair loss complicates matters even more. Always read the medication's warnings, and it is in your interest to always check with your doctor the potential side effects of any new medication that you are put on. Likewise, if you are having to take a medication for the long term and are experiencing hair loss, talk to your doctor so as to be able to know whether the hair loss is being induced by the medication or if you are suffering from MPB.

- Have blood panels performed once a year. I do this myself for optimal health, and it will allow you to build up a log of how your body is performing throughout a given time period of your life. It will also help you to potentially identify anything that is going wrong. Test your thyroid, sex hormones, glucose levels and stress hormones for a direct link to hair loss if any of these are subpar. Speak to your doctor for the best approach to perform blood tests on a yearly basis. Be aware though, it can get expensive.

Reactive:

- If you have noticed hairline recession, see a dermatologist as soon as possible. If he/she confirms MPB and you want to slow down the hair loss progression, then go on minoxidil, a drug that is almost free of side effects and that works best in the earlier stages of MPB. I must tell you, however, that there is no cure for male pattern baldness as of 2013.

- Finasteride is another proven-to-work medication, but it can have some heavy side effects in some users. I recommend you to not only see a dermatologist but also an endocrinologist if you decide to take finasteride. Get an initial blood panel measuring your hormone levels (especially levels of sex hormones), and re-test on a frequent basis as recommended by your doctor. Finasteride works by inhibiting an enzyme that converts testosterone into DHT, hence the use of finasteride should be monitored for optimal male health.

- There are other substances that may work to treat male pattern baldness, but you are best seeking the advice of a dermatologist with regards to these experimental substances. Unfortunately, many of these substances are being pushed by scammers, giving a bad image to potential substances that could work to treat MPB. Among these potentially-helpful substances are ketoconazole, saw palmetto, topical caffeine, tea tree oil, several vitamins and mineral and other natural alternatives. Do always remain skeptic of anything making wild claims; the only medications clinically-approved to treat MPB as of 2013 are minoxidil and finasteride (though dutasteride has shown great promise and may be approved at some stage).

- A hair transplant is a feasible option for those males who want to get their hair back. However, it is imperative that you research this option thoroughly because transplanting hair is a very skilled process. Furthermore, a hair transplant doesn't guarantee 100% that the transplanted hair will be MPB free, and a good hair transplant will cost thousands of dollars and will typically require more than one session.

- If you have just pulled out a chunk of hair accidentally (it will happen eventually if you grow your mane to a long length), massage the area immediately for 30 seconds, ingest 100 milligrams of vitamin C and move on. Hair that is pulled out of its follicle socket will grow back eventually, but don't make pulling out your hair a habit because repeatedly plucking your hair will damage the follicle and irreversibly halt its production of hair material (i.e. no more growth of hair strands).

- If you find yourself experiencing hair loss because you keep pulling out your hair, see a doctor. This hair-pulling habit is known as trichotillomania in the medical field and is associated with chronically-high levels of stress, anxiety and even some mental disorders. Tackling the root of the problem (no pun intended) will fix this cause of hair loss. Be aware that trichotillomania is not only limited to scalp hair, it can be manifested on other areas of the body (the eyebrow is a common area). In its most extreme form, trichotillomania will lead to bald patches in the scalp.

## A note on how overall health reflects on hair health

Listen; men live about 5 years less than women, and we go about our lives with a lot of unneeded stress and drama. Ultimately, our overall health will reflect on our hair health just as it will reflect on our sexual health or mental health.

As you have read in this chapter with regards to hair loss, this third hair issue is a condition linked with stress and hormones. A stressed body produces more cortisol, distorts its release of growth hormone and insulin, and decreases its levels of sex hormones, with all of this in unison enhancing and magnifying any hair loss taking place.

Biologically, when the body is under extreme physical or mental demands for long periods (i.e. chronic stress), it will shut down several unnecessary-to-life processes so as to remain efficient and ensure survival. Your body will prioritise your brain before your hair follicles when it is in survival mode, which is why people who are overstressed or malnourished experience dramatic hair loss and don't look good physically. On top of that, stressed people tend to be depressed, and depression is a serious health condition that will negatively impact your desire to look good including the grooming and looking after of your hair.

If you want to maximise the potential of your mane, then ensure that you are managing your life's duties and responsibilities optimally because unneeded stress will take a toll on your mane and your body. I know it is easier said than done, but many of us could start living an easier life by looking at the little things that are causing us nuisances and then removing them from our lives. And, of course, if you're going through an extremely-demanding stage of your life and can't see the light at the end of the tunnel, then do not underestimate the power of human touch and talk to someone else. Many of us males have been brainwashed to believe that looking for help when the going gets tough is emasculating, when the reverse is actually true: a real man will always aim to maximise the tools available to him (people/sources of help) so as to live a better life!

## **Conclusion**

Over the long term, you will be facing 3 issues with regards to your mane: dry hair, tangled hair and hair loss. To battle these issues, you must have a set of measures that are continuously implemented, with these measures making up one part of your hair-care strategy (the other part being your nutrition).

Dry hair and tangled hair are 2 issues that will just about be taken care of via your hair grooming. However, the specific implementing of certain hair-care measures concerning these 2 issues will bulletproof your hair, and, what's just as good, these measures will fit conveniently into your lifestyle as a male.

With regards to hair loss, it is male pattern baldness (MPB) that is most important to us males. This condition is treated with 2 medications, but we currently have no permanent cure for MPB. Likewise, proper intake of nutrients (to be covered in the next chapter) plus paying more attention to your daily interaction with your hair will ensure that you extend the life of your locks.

Lastly, proper stress management throughout your lifetime is imperative in order to keep your hair strands healthy. You want to have the best-looking mane possible, which means that you must remove unneeded sources of stress from your life so as to maximise the optimal health potential of your body and, by default, of your hair.

# Anthony's barbershop case study

Mario was a 35-year old surfer who had come to Anthony with the biggest dead rat you could possibly imagine. Mario had long straight hair that was very dry as he had no clue about hair care or hair grooming. Moreover, he had a tendency to tie his hair very tight into a ponytail which had caused his hairline to recede. Upon enquiring, Mario told Anthony that he (Mario) had indeed noticed his hairline receding a bit but that he wasn't sure as his long hair was masking any scalp changes he could be experiencing.

Anthony quickly walked Mario through the optimal hair-grooming aspect and told him about the hair-care measures to battle his dry hair. It was fairly obvious that Mario needed to find out his optimal shampooing frequency (he shampooed his hair twice daily!) and that he needed to insert a normal conditioner as well as a deep conditioner in there. Furthermore, Mario was advised by Anthony on the right way to tie a ponytail (i.e. release tension from the tied hair), and he was also told to visit a dermatologist about his hairline as Mario had shown an interest in knowing whether he was balding or not.

Mario came back to Anthony's barbershop 3 weeks later and he had good news. He had started using the generic hair-grooming routine (as covered in the previous chapter) and was working on finding out his optimal shampooing frequency. His mane was looking much, much better, and he had instantly noticed an improvement from the deep conditioner that Anthony had recommended Mario to use on the day after his previous visit (Mario's hair was that dry!). Furthermore, it turns out that a dermatologist was able to confirm to Mario that he wasn't suffering MPB; however, Mario had caused some tremendous damage to his hairline from leaving his hair constantly tied too tight; luckily for him though, Anthony had advised Mario to release tension from the ponytail and Mario had started using this measure so as to ensure that he wasn't worsening the traction alopecia already manifested on his hairline. After 6 weeks, Mario's hair looked, literally, as if it were brand new.

# 5) Hair-Care Aspect: Eating Right For Great-Looking Hair

You may have heard before the saying "you are what you eat". While I don't wholeheartedly agree with this cliché, I have seen on myself and on others what optimal nutrition can do to one's hair and even life. From better hair to a better body to an overall better life, your nutrition should be optimised to cater to your lifestyle as a 21$^{st}$ century male.

"Organic", "fat-free", "Atkins diet", "free of preservatives", "no-carb pizza" or "aspartame" are just some of the fancy words that we get bombarded with every day. For the most part, we don't know what they are or what they really mean, and unfortunately we have to live with the fact that many companies and people out there take advantage of semantic boundaries and wrongful associations. Organic food is twice as expensive as non-organic food, yet being organic doesn't guarantee it to be healthier or diet friendly as many people wrongfully think of organic foods. Likewise, low-fat products are not necessarily healthier than their regular counterparts, and, many times, the fat content of the former is substituted by adding lots of sugar and other just as unhealthy ingredients (e.g. high-fructose corn syrup) to mask the food's otherwise bland taste. In fact, next time that you are in the supermarket, go to the dairy section and read the ingredients of the flashiest and most-colourful low-fat yoghurt that you can find on display, and see this nutritional dichotomy for yourself.

Over the years, I have found that whatever diet I chose that improved my health also had the side effect of improving my hair. The body is a perfect machine relying on homeostasis and biological harmony, hence a change in one bodily process will have a knock-on effect on other bodily processes, and thus the need to see one's diet as a way to improve one's health and body as a whole and, by default, one's hair. What's more is that an optimal diet and nutritional approach will not only improve the looks of your locks but also ensure that your hair remains atop your head for a long time.

Your hair follicles are alive, and, for them to produce hair, they need optimal nutrition as well as blood flow to deliver the right nutrients. Your hair follicles are dug in your skin, the latter (skin) being the largest organ in the body, so a lot of internal processes are going on to allow the hair follicles to continue to produce hair material (i.e. hair strands) non-stop. Thus, while throwing exotic ingredients on your hair strands in the hopes that your hair can breathe more oxygen or can live happily is an exercise in futility, there is certainly quite a merit and good sense in trying to get optimal nutrients delivered to your hair follicles endogenously (i.e. via your diet and nutritional approach).

There is no one-and-only nutritional approach to making your hair look its best. In my case, the nutritional approach that I have used successfully, and which I will share with you, is one that I have found to allow for optimal sebum secretion, a healthy scalp, stronger and thicker hair strands, and is one that has also helped me to avoid excessive hair shedding or being hit by male pattern baldness. The aforementioned benefits brought by my optimal nutritional approach have greatly promoted the good looks and optimal health of my mane, and, so far, it has allowed me to secure my hair for the long term as I have paired my nutritional approach with a solid set of proactive and reactive hair-care measures (i.e. my tailored hair-care strategy).

There are a lot of diets out there and plenty of nutritional approaches that one can follow. Through my experience, I have found a positive correlation between my overall health and the health of my hair: whenever my health was at its peak via my nutritional approach, so was my hair's health. Thus, the nutritional approach that I follow is my 1 stone to kill 2 juicy birds: optimal overall health and optimal hair health.

What is a nutritional approach? That which comprises everything you ingest, from the foods you eat (i.e. diet) to the nutritional supplements you may so take, altogether providing you with macronutrients (protein, carbohydrates and fats) and micronutrients (vitamins, minerals and other essential nutrients) that are used by the body to support its functioning and to maintain your health and well-being. In the context of this book, your nutritional approach is made up of your diet and your nutritional supplementation (the latter being optional).

When it comes to your diet, you should not be seeing it as a short-term change in your nutritional habits in order to lose weight or look better. Instead, your diet should be integrated into a nutritional approach seeking optimal health above all as, in turn, such a diet will enhance your hair and image. This has been exactly my case, which is why I want to include and share in this chapter my nutritional approach to maximise the health of your hair so that you can thus learn about an indispensable element to having great hair that is overlooked by the majority of men desiring better hair.

The diet that I follow is high in protein intake, low in carbohydrate intake and moderate in fat intake. After years of experimenting with different ratios of these 3 macronutrients (protein:carbohydrates:fats), I have found such "high protein:low carbohydrate:moderate fat" diet to be the best for me and for my hair. I also try to eat as close to natural as possible, so I always choose the least-processed and man-modified food items, which automatically ensures that I get the most amount of nutrients from the foods I eat. An example of this would be orange juice: instead of buying a pack of processed orange juice from the supermarket shelf, I will instead buy oranges in their natural state and then make the orange juice myself. I apply this very principle to my diet and when I buy food; that way I am guaranteed to maximise the food that I eat from both a nutritional and economical perspective.

I have not only seen this on myself but on others too: a diet composed of a high protein, low carbohydrate and moderate fat intake, together with a natural and unprocessed food emphasis is the best dietary option to safeguard one's mane over the long term. My hair has looked its best with a diet like this one, and I have been able to notice the changes in the health and looks of my hair when I have gone back to using such a diet at different points in my lifetime. If we consider this diet's documented health benefits and the huge anecdotal evidence that can be found online vouching for a natural and unprocessed diet, it then leaves no doubt that a diet similar to mine is a great addition for the health-conscious modern male who wants to achieve and maintain a great head of Is, Ss, Es or Zs.

It is thus that I would like to give you the insight to my diet and nutritional approach so that you can learn from what has worked for me and then be able to apply some of my nutritional principles and tactics to your particular case. As a cautionary note, I must warn you that you should at all times consult a doctor before embarking on a diet regimen (including mine) or doing anything that may affect your health in one way or another. Your health should always come first no matter what, so first consult with your doctor if you decide to change your dietary habits or emulate my personal experience with my nutritional approach for optimal hair health.

# My diet

I only eat once or twice a day on average. I prefer to avoid spiking my insulin levels frequently because I don't like the consequent fluctuations in blood sugar levels. I feel that my optimal energy levels are best achieved with fasting for the most part of my day, and I prefer to enjoy 1 or 2 big meals instead of snacking throughout the day.

I also stick to certain food groups that I have found to be the essentials for overall health and hair health. I reward myself with eating whatever I want once every 1 or 2 weeks (i.e. a cheat day); I'll do this typically on a Friday or Saturday as this is when it is most convenient for a social life. I prefer not to obsess about breaking my diet, and I will break my diet if the occasion calls for it, then making up for it by either exercising more or delaying the next cheat day. Regardless, 90% of my time is spent either fasted or eating from the food groups below:

- Meat: lean cuts and from the butcher. I avoid processed meat for the most part. Steak and chicken breast make a big chunk of my meat intake, and I love eating them. I also gulp down whole chickens often, there is just something primitive and manly about devouring 2 whole chickens with your hands in one sitting. I throw in some vegetables with the 2 chickens for an added healthy touch (cavemen also ate their veggies). High-quality protein is of the utmost value to grow strong hair strands, and meat (be it red or white) provides high quantities of high-quality protein as well as hair-friendly micronutrients such as zinc and several B vitamins.

- Oily fish: I eat salmon or sardines at least once a week. Canned sardines are my favourite and despite their light processing to fit inside the can, they still remain very nutritious and are very tasty in extra-virgin olive oil. With salmon, I prefer to oven cook it or fry it lightly with slow heat. The precious nutrients that I seek in oily fish are omega-3 fatty acids, which are essential fats needed for optimal sebum production. Most oily fishes also contain vitamin A, which is an excellent skin moisturiser and sustains optimal skin cell production (i.e. optimises the health of your hair follicles).

- Dairy: I love cheese, and I eat cheese regularly. I prefer the unpasteurised type because it is made with raw milk (less processing): good Manchego (Spanish),

Parmesan (Italian) and Emmental (Swiss) cheeses are made with unpasteurised milk and taste great. I also eat a good amount of cottage cheese and yoghurt; I don't drink much milk because I find that it gives me too much stomach discomfort if I drink more than 2 pints. Dairy is another excellent source of high-quality protein and also provides many hair-friendly vitamins including vitamin A and the many Bs.

• Eggs: I call eggs "nature's multivitamin". They are a staple in my diet, and I strive to eat 2 to 6 whole eggs per day. After experimenting with different quantities, I have found a relatively-high daily consumption of eggs to have absolutely no negative effect on my cholesterol levels. Eggs have so many nutrients that are essential to male health (including hair health) that leaving them out of one's diet should be regarded as nutritional suicide. They are also cheap and multifunctional, and I eat them mostly boiled or scrambled.

• Fruits: I base most of my fruit intake around berries and water-dense fruits such as pomegranates and kiwis. They are packed with a wide array of nutrients and antioxidants not found elsewhere in nature, so I consider these fruits essential to optimal health and hair.

• Vegetables: I go through pounds of leafy vegetables every week, and I eat most leafy veggies. I also eat tomatoes, cucumbers and onions every day, and I make salads with all of these plus the leafy vegetables. I do not eat starchy vegetables except for the occasional beetroot. Most vegetables contain ample amounts of hair-essential vitamin C and antioxidants.

• Water: I drink tap water except if I am living in a country with bad-quality tap water (e.g. Dubai). I drink about 3 litres of water per day and go through an extra 3 litres in each weightlifting session that I carry out. I find that most people, including myself, overeat when they are thirsty because the body activates the hunger cue so as to obtain water from food sources since it is not getting it from liquid sources. Sipping water throughout the day is a great way to kill any unneeded hunger pangs, and I have a big glass of water sitting next to me as I type these words. Adequate and daily internal hydration (i.e.

drinking water) is indispensable to life, including skin health (and by default your hair follicles).

- Oils: I only use extra-virgin olive oil for cooking and dressing because not only is this oil resistant to heat but it is also packed with vitamin E and monounsaturated fat, so this particular oil doesn't alter my intake ratio of omega-3:omega-6 fatty acids (as opposed to how sunflower oil would do). Despite being the most expensive of oils, I always buy extra-virgin olive oil from Spain since southern Spain has the best region in the world to grow olives, and the olive oil from there is magnificent. Always go "extra-virgin" because it is the least refined (processed) of oils and contains the highest levels of vitamin E, a vitamin that behaves as an antioxidant in the body and that has a skin-enhancing effect.

- Nuts: at least once a week, I eat a blend of almonds, pecan nuts and walnuts. Just like with extra-virgin olive oil, nuts are a great source of vitamin E and are tasty. I like to use them in salads because they make salads taste great and you can get creative with them. Since vitamin E is a liposoluble vitamin (i.e. the body stores it), you don't need to eat nuts every day: once or twice a week is sufficient for a hair-friendly intake of vitamin E.

- Fats: I also use butter from milk as well as extra-virgin coconut butter for my cooking. The butter I use is from cows that have grazed in grass since grass-fed cows produce higher-quality milk. I buy extra-virgin coconut butter because not only is it great for hair as a hairstyling agent but also because it is a great cooking butter if I decide to cook something exotic. Butter contains vitamin A, which is the big daddy of hair-friendly micronutrients.

- Iodised salt: I use iodised salt because most foods lack in iodine. Iodine is a nutrient that is of the utmost importance for the proper functioning of the thyroid gland. A low intake of iodine in the body will manifest as hair loss and brittle hair, apart from causing other hypothyroid-like symptoms. Iodised salt is an excellent way to fulfil one's daily intake of iodine.

All of the above foods are what I would eat on a weekly basis. I pick and rotate them daily so as to meet my macronutrient and micronutrient needs and have variety in my diet. My fridge is always full of these food items, and I try to avoid precooked food because I want to know what I am putting in my mouth.

## My nutritional supplementation

While I don't always use nutritional supplements, I like to use them frequently so as to complement my diet and bulletproof my nutritional approach. On a daily basis, I typically add the following nutrients in the form of supplements to my diet:

- Calcium

- Magnesium

- Zinc

- Copper

- Vitamin B complex

- Multivitamin with 100% of the Reference Daily Intake (RDI)

- Vitamin C with rose hips

- Cod liver oil (very rich in vitamin A and D)

The above supplement regimen is just the icing on the cake to my diet, and the 2 together (diet plus supplementation) make my nutritional approach. I already get enough macronutrients and micronutrients from my diet, so the daily doses that I use for my supplements are taken into consideration with what I am going to be eating for the day. If I am going to be eating 2 pounds of steak, there is no need for me to take zinc, or if I am going to be ingesting considerable amounts of dairy, I will skip the calcium (or only take a minimal amount).

There are other supplements around that I have used in the past and have helped towards better hair, but these are the ones that I take consistently and have been of long-term benefit to my hair as well as overall heath.

# The keys to my nutritional approach

As you have been able to read from the diet that I use to look after my hair, my diet is high in protein, low in carbohydrates and moderate in fat intake, and it is based around nutrient-dense natural foods. My diet is rich in protein and contains a good source of natural fats; I do not get my fat intake from fast foods, and I instead get my intake from natural foods while emphasising an optimal ratio of omega-3:omega-6 essential fatty acids (1:2 is good for me). I avoid food that has been processed heavily, and I allow myself for infrequent meal treats. Moreover, I use nutritional supplements to complement my diet and not the other way around.

If I were to boil down my nutritional approach to 6 essential points, I would go with the following personal observations for a great head of hair:

1. Take in an adequate amount of protein

While the Reference Daily Intake (RDI) for protein for an adult male is easy to achieve (it's about 60 grams), I always take in more and strive to hit 0.8 grams per pound of body weight. That means that if my body weight is 200lbs, I will ingest about 160 grams of protein per day, sometimes even going higher or lower than that. I must note that I engage in heavy strength training, and an increased protein intake is suitable for strength athletes. However, I have experimented with taking lower quantities of protein (including only the established RDI), and I have found not only my training recovery impaired but also the health of my hair (most notably, a weaker tensile strength of the hair strands). From my experiments and findings, 0.8 grams per pound of body weight is my perfect number for hair health.

Remember that protein contains the building blocks for hair, so you certainly don't want to be malnourished in this macronutrient. The RDI is the bare minimum for an adult male, and I have found a higher intake of protein than that of the established RDI to yield stronger hair strands. A daily protein intake of 0.6 grams per pound of body weight is the lowest amount from which I have noticed a positive effect on my hair, whether it was during a period of my life in which I was weightlifting or whether it was during a period in which I didn't lift heavy weights. Likewise, other men who have followed my advice in the past have reported back that 0.6 grams per pound of bodyweight is also their minimal number to grow strong hair strands.

From my experience and findings, a daily protein intake of 0.6 grams per pound of body weight is an optimal one for sedentary individuals who want better hair while a higher daily intake (over 0.8 g/lbs) is better suited for those who engage in any form of frequent weight training. Make sure to consult your doctor first before increasing your protein intake as this nutritional point can only be done if your body is healthy (e.g. healthy kidneys).

2. Increase your fish oil intake

While increasing your intake of fish oil is a great action (i.e. part of the strategy) for optimal hair health, it is not always reasonable to be eating fish every day. First, not every fish has adequate amounts of oils, one needs to eat oily fish such as salmon, sardines or the liver of cod fish. Second, there is a risk of ingesting too much mercury from eating the bigger types of fish too frequently (e.g. shark or swordfish). Mercury is a chemical element that accumulates through the food chain, meaning that the biggest of sea predators will have the highest levels of mercury in their meat.

Fish oil contains an awesome-mane-friendly type of fats: omega-3. Omega-3 is the name for a bunch of essential fatty acids that enhance optimal sebum production and secretion and that most of us males don't ingest enough of. Omega-3 fatty acids are essential for the proper functioning of the body, so lacking in their intake will manifest itself physically. If you are not taking in optimal levels of omega-3s, your hair will be brittle and frizzy, and you will not be maximising your own sebum via the Sebum Coating method.

I have found that 3 grams of omega-3 fatty acids per day is excellent for my hair. While achieving this intake through food alone is doable, supplements in the form of fish-oil gel capsules are extremely convenient. On top of that, the best fish-oil brands ensure the removal of any toxic pollutants that could be found in the extracted oil itself, so with supplements you get your optimal intake of fish oil in a convenient manner while avoiding exposure to mercury and other toxic elements.

Lastly, most vegetable oils and fats (especially ones used for cooking) contain too much omega-6 fatty acids and too little omega-3 fatty acids, and it is the balance of your "omega-3:omega-6" intake ratio that matters especially for cardiovascular health and inflammation in the body (male pattern baldness is thought to be partially mediated via chronic inflammation in the scalp). Thus, it is imperative that you get omega-3 fatty acids in your diet so as to balance said omega 3:omega 6 intake ratio. Ideally, you want to have a ratio of 1:2 (or even 1:1), and a typical pro-disease Western diet is 1:15.

3. <u>Vitamin A is king for a healthy scalp</u>

I first experienced the benefits of vitamin A on my scalp while experimenting with fish oil. I had been recording the results of a few trials I had done with fish oil supplements when I decided to give cod liver oil some 8 weeks of trialling. Cod liver oil is a specific type of fish oil that is extremely rich in vitamin A. Most conventional fish oil supplements have trivial amounts of vitamin A whereas cod liver oil not only offers a great source of omega-3 fatty acids but it is also one of nature's best sources of vitamin A (and vitamin D too).

While my notes showed a noticeable benefit from fish oil on how healthy and shiny my locks looked, when I trialled cod liver oil I also noticed a much lower rate of skin flaking (i.e. shedding dead skin cells). During these experiments, I was sporting my mane in a High and Tight Recon on purpose since this hairstyle allowed me to keep the sides and back of my head shaved and thus be able to document any changes in scalp health.

With cod liver oil, I noticed a scalp benefit that I didn't notice with fish oil. I was shaving my scalp every 2 days, and every time that I would shave my hair during the cod liver oil trial, the shaved scalp would not become irritated and red. On the other hand, every time that I shaved my scalp when I was taking fish oil alone, I would experience mild irritation from the razor, and the skin would turn a light red for a few hours. Once I finished the trial with cod liver oil, I decided to continue using fish oil, but I also started taking vitamin A at a dose equating the dose ingested during the cod liver oil trial, and, lo and behold, I experienced the same anti-irritation and skin-smoothing benefit of cold liver oil! Vitamin A has been known for decades to be nature's skin moisturiser and is a vitamin that is highly underrated.

Bear in mind that the scalp contains the thriving part of your hair; the scalp contains the follicles that continuously produce new hair material. A healthy scalp contains, by default, healthy hair follicles, which in turn equates healthy hair strands (i.e. glossier and stronger); this is why your hair-care strategy must target the hair follicles too, not just the hair strands. Vitamin A is one of the best vitamins to use to notice a boost in hair quality starting from the very root (pun intended).

If you want to use cod liver oil, be aware that it tastes even worse than plain fish oil, so you are better off buying gel caps instead of the liquid. Also, be aware that cod liver oil is very rich in vitamin D, and you should consult your doctor prior to using cod liver oil as your own skin makes vitamin D when exposed to sunlight, hence using cod liver oil may push your vitamin D levels to higher than desired for optimal health. Furthermore, fish oil (including cod liver oil) can anticoagulate your blood when taken in very high doses or if taken when anticoagulation medication is being used (e.g. warfarin).

If you choose not to use cod liver oil, make sure that you are ingesting optimal amounts of other vitamin A-rich sources such as eggs, beef liver and dairy. Lastly, if you go down the supplement route, buy vitamin A in the form of retinol and not beta-carotene as the former is much stronger than the latter.

4. <u>Whole eggs are superfoods</u>

I view whole eggs as superfoods. They are choked with essential vitamins and minerals, and they even contain some omega-3 fatty acids. Eggs are an excellent source of protein and sulphur, the latter being a mineral associated with stronger hair strands. Moreover, eggs can be a staple food for those who don't eat meat since many of the essential micronutrients in meat are also found in eggs.

With eggs, I have noticed a special benefit in terms of the strength of my hair. Since eggs are nature's multivitamin, my hair has looked great every time that my egg intake was higher than what most men ingest (4+ whole eggs per day). Call me, perhaps, a good responder to eggs, but I have always found my hair and body strength to be at its peak when I was eating eggs in abundance.

Scientists have found out in the laboratory that most nutrients are best absorbed and best utilised when they are ingested as they are found in nature. Calcium is a perfect example, the fat naturally found in milk enhances the absorption of calcium, which makes milk a superior source of calcium than calcium supplements alone. Thus, I would not be surprised if, with eggs, the synergies of all the nutrients in the yolk and the albumen yielded a superior form of hair-optimising nutrients such as protein, fatty acids, sulphur and vitamin A.

Again, if you are going to emulate my high consumption of eggs, consult a doctor first because you may end up negatively affecting your cholesterol levels.

5. Berries and fruits for those antioxidants

Not only are fruits nature's tasty desserts but many fruits are also great sources of antioxidants, vitamins and nutrients that are not found anywhere else in nature. I am a huge fan of berries in their culinary (not botanical) definition: blueberries, strawberries, raspberries and redberries are my favourites although, if I had to pick one, I'd go with blueberries because they are a packed with huge amounts of antioxidants. Blueberries are tasty, can be used to make smoothies and milk shakes, can be sprinkled on pretty much anything, and they have an excellent nutrient profile.

While the tangible hair benefit from eating berries hasn't been as pronounced as the hair benefit from ingesting fish oil and vitamin A, I have certainly found a great hair benefit from complementing my diet with extra vitamin C, a vitamin found in vast amounts in all berries. Many times, it is the lack of certain nutrients in one's diet that leads to tangible and noticeable negative effects on one's hair, and, with blueberries in my diet, I do know for sure that my vitamin C intake is more than satisfied.

As I've mentioned in the previous point, nutrients are best utilised by the body as they are found in nature, so the vitamin C found in berries is highly useful and efficiently absorbed for our hair-optimising purposes. Thus, strive to often ingest fruits and especially berries, for you will be building with these the foundation to a nutritional approach that is excellent in its micronutrient intake.

6. Use of nutritional supplements as a complement to your diet

Also known as food supplements or dietary supplements, nutritional supplements do absolutely have a place in one's nutritional approach. You cannot always ensure that you are getting the highest amounts of nutrients from the foods you eat, so nutritional supplements allow you to bulletproof your diet and overall nutrition. The problem is that many men think of nutritional supplements as magic pills that, when taken in excess, will lead to whatever it is that the supplement's manufacturer claims. Not only is thinking of nutritional supplements as magic pills a waste of your time but their excessive intake may also prove dangerous or counterproductive. To use nutritional supplements the right way, you should research them first and use them to complement your diet so as to create an optimal nutritional approach.

While there are many nutritional supplements that may be somewhat beneficial to your hair and hair growth, the following nutritional supplements are those that are of great use exclusively for your hair-bettering efforts:

- Zinc (taken with copper in a 10:1 ratio)

- Vitamin A, D and E (taken separately or together and preferably with a meal)

- The whole spectrum of the B vitamins, especially biotin (vitamin B7)

- Vitamin C with citrus flavonoids

- Iodine as a supplement alone or in the form of iodised salt or kelp

- Fish oil or cod liver oil

- Methylsulfonylmethane (MSM)

- A multivitamin with 100% of the RDI for all vitamins and minerals

- Whey protein if you find that you cannot meet your optimal intake of protein via food alone

All of the above when taken as nutritional supplements and when added to an optimal diet will lead to better hair. Any time that you want to introduce a supplement into your nutritional approach, make sure that you research it thoroughly and that you consult your doctor before; some nutritional supplements may actually lead to micronutrient deficiencies or may accumulate beyond safe levels, so tread carefully. My advice is to obtain 100% of the RDI for all vitamins and minerals via supplementation so that you bulletproof your nutritional approach without risking toxic levels of micronutrients.

## Conclusion

Optimal nutrition is imperative to make the most of your hair. By providing the essential building blocks to your hair endogenously, you ensure that your hair grows healthy, strong and will have its lifetime extended. You provide these nutrients endogenously via your nutritional approach, which is made up of your diet and your nutritional supplementation.

As modern males, our diets are lacking in nutrients, thus it's in your interest to look at your current diet and identify where it may be lacking in nutrients. Protein, omega-3s, vitamin A, Bs, C and E, zinc and iodine are among those nutrients that need to be taken daily either via your diet or your supplementation in order to achieve the optimal health of your hair.

Your nutritional approach is one part of your hair-care strategy; the other part to your hair-care strategy consists of your hair-care measures for the Big 3 (as per the previous chapter). You must now come up with you own strategy based on the studying of this chapter and the previous chapter because your own hair-care measures and nutritional approach need to be customised to your current case.

Once you come up with your hair-care strategy, you will have fulfilled the hair-care aspect of your hair-management equation. Since you will have already optimised your hair-grooming and hair-profiling aspects before going on to optimise your hair-care aspect, you will be in a position, as you customise your hair-care strategy, that will allow you to truly make the most of your hair-management equation and thus of your own locks!

## Anthony's barbershop case study

Terry was a successful business owner who used to come to Anthony's barbershop frequently. Anthony had noticed over the last few months that Terry's wavy hair had gone from looking great and healthy to being brittle and losing its healthy looks. Anthony and I had talked many times before of the importance of nutrition for having great-looking hair, so Anthony knew something was up when, one day, he examined Terry's hair prior to giving him a haircut.

As Anthony gave Terry his usual haircut, Anthony asked Terry about any changes to his diet as of lately. Terry told Anthony that, over the last 3 months, he had gone through an overly-stressing period because his business was taking off hugely and he needed to be 24/7 over the business so as to support its growth. Terry confessed to Anthony that his diet had taken a hit and that he (Terry) knew that his diet was very poor. Terry had gone from eating healthy (he was a fitness enthusiast) to ordering takeaway food that consisted of pizzas and garbage food. His diet had changed drastically, and it showed in his hair.

Terry had already been planning to fix his diet before visiting Anthony on that same day. However, it was in this aforementioned day, during the timespan of Terry's haircut, that Anthony and Terry talked at length about fixing his (Terry's) diet and introducing a few nutritional supplements. Terry was still enduring the highly-stressing period related to his business, so he had to still rely on takeaway food. However, Anthony recommended Terry to, instead of ordering pizza, order food that consisted primarily of protein: whole chickens, steak and low-fat hamburgers. Furthermore, Anthony recommended Terry to introduce the 4 hair-friendly vitamins (A, Bs, C and E) as well as fish oil and to up his zinc intake.

Some 6 weeks later, Terry came back for another haircut and, voila, his hair looked much better. Because Terry liked to have his hair cut short (½ inch), the new hair growth (6 week's worth of) was very visible and Anthony could actually discern where the new hair growth started from the difference in looks within the same hair strands! Terry asked Anthony to cut his hair so that only the previous 6 week's growth would be visible and, after the haircut was finished, Terry looked like a new man with his new healthy head of Ss.

# 6) Giving Your Mane Its Shape: Hairstyles, Hair Accessories, Straightening Your Locks, Growing That Mane And Getting A Haircut

This chapter deals with the hairstyles available to you once you have optimised your hair-management equation. Your chosen hairstyle (also spelled hair style) is part of your hair-grooming routine, but you must first set up the basis of your hair-grooming routine as indicated in the hair-grooming chapter so as to be able to make the most of any hairstyles you may so choose. In fact, you can choose to not put your hair into a hairstyle per se, for your hair will be looking great anyway as you will still have optimised the hair-grooming aspect of your hair-management equation. Remember, get your hair-grooming routine sorted out, optimise the hair-grooming stages, get your routine down to a few minutes, and then, only then, worry about putting your hair into whatever hairstyles.

When it comes to the hairstyles, it is imperative for you to know which you can choose according to your hair type and hair length; what is feasible for kinky hair is not feasible for straight hair and vice versa. Moreover, many males make the mistake of thinking that the hairstyles that they see in magazines can be adapted to their own particular case, when nothing could be further from the truth: hairstyles done in photo shoots for magazines are many times performed with wigs, are airbrushed and are also photoshopped. Furthermore, having a subpar hair-grooming routine and hair-care strategy will make achieving most hairstyles impossible; your hair needs to be properly looked after to be able to respond its best to any styling you want to do. Thus, it is once you get your hair grooming and hair care sorted that the rest, including hairstyles, will flow naturally.

It is very important to be realistic about what hairstyles can and cannot be done on your hair. Whatever your hair type may be, you have styling options available, so don't worry about the flashy hairstyles that you see in magazines and that make you feel bad about your own locks because you can't copy those uber/trendy/fabulous (insert hip word) hairstyles. What truly matters is that you know how to look after your hair day in and day out as well as for the rest of your life, which then enables you to have great-looking hair regardless of the hairstyle you choose to sport.

# Haircut vs. Hairstyle

Before we go into the hairstyles that I recommend for each hair type, it is imperative that you are aware of the difference between a haircut and a hairstyle, for these terms tend to be confused and misinterpreted by many guys.

As it goes, to rock a certain hairstyle you first need the proper haircut. Many of us, myself included, have made the mistake of using both terms interchangeably despite each conveying something different. Sure, they both relate to hair, but a "haircut" involves cutting while a "hairstyle" involves styling. I want you to be sure of the meaning of each because, for your hair-bettering efforts, you will sooner or later get a haircut and try a hairstyle.

## Haircut

A haircut refers to the specific act of trimming or cutting the hair so that it is given a shape. It is done in the moment and can be regarded as part of a routine to cut the length of the hair every so often, or it can be done with a specific cosmetic goal in mind (e.g. give the hair a certain shape for a hairstyle you have in mind). A haircut is commonly done with scissors (aka shears) and/or a hair clipper. An example of a haircut is a buzz cut: cropping the hair to a very short length all around the head and performed with a hair clipper.

## Hairstyle

This refers to the modification and manipulation of the hair without cutting it so that it looks in a certain form or shape. Having said that, a hairstyle can also be regarded as the final hair shape obtained after a haircut as the shape obtained is the one desired to be worn daily until the next haircut. With men, a hairstyle is most commonly thought of in the long term; that is, a hairstyle would be worn for weeks or months at a time according to the preference of the individual although a hairstyle can also be worn for a single or specific occasion. Some common hairstyles include the Afro (kinky hair) or the Side Swept (wavy hair).

As it relates to your efforts, you go to the barber to get a haircut and you give yourself a hairstyle every morning after you get out of the shower to implement the third stage of your hair-grooming routine. You can get a haircut done to specifically sport a hairstyle, or you can simply go for a haircut every number of weeks to keep your hair at a certain length. Likewise, you can also give yourself a haircut instead of going to the barber although I recommend you to only do this if you truly master the art of cutting hair and, even then, limit it to giving yourself small trims as you run the risk of ruining your hair in an instant (I speak from experience!).

Hairstyles are typically done in the bathroom as part of your daily hair grooming after you are done with the conditioning stage and approach the styling stage. However, you can give yourself a hairstyle under other scenarios not requiring the previous two stages of the hair-grooming routine; all you have to bear in mind is to always dampen your hair prior to styling it: never give yourself a hairstyle on non-damp hair as that is a recipe for disaster, though you can retouch the hairstyle without having to dampen your hair again.

## Hairstyles for hair types

It is imperative for you to know that not all hairstyles will be suitable for your particular hair type. I am not here to sell you dreams; that is not my job. Unless you love spending much of your free time in hair salons having your hair retouched while drinking tea and discussing the latest Hollywood gossip with your hairstylist, you should then stick to those hairstyles that suit your hair type. Absolutely every hair type can be styled with cool and suitable hairstyles; you just need to know which ones are feasible for your specific hair type.

I recommend you to go for the simpler and more convenient hairstyles; basically, go for those hairstyles that are easy to stay with and that you can give yourself in a moment. Elaborate hairstyles look great in magazines and photo shoots, but they are not convenient for most men because they involve great investments in time and effort, not to mention money as you will have to be frequently visiting the hair salon to keep the chosen hairstyle looking neat. Of course, for once-in-a-while occasions, feel free to go nuts with elaborate hairstyles if that's what you want, but do not make them a daily thing because your newly-acquired hair-grooming routine has a convenience factor that is shot down with elaborate hairstyles.

While you will find below a plethora of hairstyles to choose from, I advise you to first consider the beautifully-simple Shake & Go hairstyle as a starting point to experimenting with hairstyles on your hair.

The Shake & Go hairstyle is done by making your hair damp (e.g. after a shower), coating the locks with whichever hairstyling agent you decide to go with and then shaking your head briefly to allow the hair to sit on top of your head freely. Your Is, Ss, Es or Zs will just sit there, showing their natural form and looking awesome, provided that you have already mastered your hair-grooming routine and hair-care strategy. The Shake & Go is a favourite hairstyle of mine, and it works well with all hair types especially when the hair is at a medium length.

The cool thing about starting with the Shake & Go hairstyle before venturing into the rest of hairstyles available is that you will get to know how your particular hair type reacts, adapts and expresses with the hairstyling agent you use. If you try the Shake & Go hairstyle for a week, you will be able to learn how your hair reacts without being manipulated and you'll familiarise yourself with the Damp vs. Dry effect, with all of this then paving the way for optimally choosing further hairstyles. Moreover, the Shake & Go hairstyle is suitable for all types of hair and will never let you down during those times when you just can't be bothered to choose a hairstyle for the day and want something fast and aesthetic.

What follows are my recommended hairstyles for each hair type and hair length. By all means, they are not the only ones available for each of the 4 hair types, and you can try the hairstyles that I recommend for the hair types that precede and follow your particular type (e.g. if you have coiled hair, you can try the hairstyles recommended for wavy and kinky hair). The recommended hairstyles that you will now be finding for your specific hair type will, however, suit you optimally.

## Straight hair

Straight hair is the least difficult of all hair types to style. If you have this hair type, you won't have much of an issue with your hair looking different between damp and dry states, so you can do most hairstyles knowing that your hair will still look the same at the end of the day as it did at the start of the day when it was styled. Wax, pomades, hair gel and mousse are the hairstyling agents that will work great for styling your mane.

- Spikes (short length)

This hairstyle is very popular among males, and it revolves around lifting one's hair to create the illusion of spikes. Use hair gel to lift your locks up, and, once you have lifted them all, use your fingers to go lock by lock to further define their spike shape, rapidly running the fingers from mid-length to the tip so as to ensure that all locks are coated with hair gel. You can do all the hair on your head or only do the spikes on the top of your head. You can coat the tips of the spikes with hair wax too so they look moulded.

A perfect example of the Spikes hairstyle is Taylor Lautner's hair from The Twilight Saga films.

- The Shaggy (medium length)

The Shaggy hairstyle (aka Shag) is one that aims to emulate an out-of-bed messy look, hence it is great for medium-length straight hair. For this hairstyle, you will need a hair dryer: coat your hair previously with hair mousse and then blow-dry your hair as you run your fingers through your hair to create a messy look by tousling the locks. Additionally, once the hair has been blow-dried, coat your fingers with some more hair mousse and run your fingers again through your hair, this time giving a bit of direction to your hair as desired, but always abiding by the "messy look" concept.

British singer Rod Stewart has sported the Shaggy hairstyle throughout his 50s and can still be seen sporting a Shag despite nearing his 70th birthday!

- The Side Fringe (medium length)

With this hairstyle, you will part your hair from either the left or right temple. You will have the front of your hair covering your forehead (i.e. fringe) and styled in your desired direction. You choose how much you want the fringe to cover your forehead. Use a conventional or wide-tooth comb and run it smoothly through the locks as you part them to the side and set the fringe on your forehead. Try to use the smallest amount of your chosen hairstyling agent on the fringe so as to avoid getting the product on your forehead; your fringe will hold up in place with little product.

The Side Fringe is best exemplified in the movie <u>17 Again</u> by Zac Efron.

- <u>The Shoulder Length (long length)</u>

This hairstyle involves growing your mane to reach the shoulders or base of the neck. It requires the hair to be trimmed in layers so that all of it reaches the shoulders and doesn't exceed this length mark. For your hair type, the hair at the very top of your head will require an extended length of about 12 inches to reach the shoulders whereas the hair at the nape will only need about 4 inches of extended length, hence the need to trim the hair in layers as it grows.

You are best growing the Shoulder Length hairstyle by first getting a haircut that has all your hair at an even length all around your head so that you start growing your Is from the same length. Then, trim the hair as each segment of the scalp reaches the shoulders.

The Shoulder Length is a favourite hairstyle of Johnny Depp in between filming movies (he grows his straight locks out to shoulder length then cuts them again for another movie).

## Wavy hair

Because wavy hair doesn't tend to coil and, instead, expresses itself in a wave-like pattern, the Damp vs Dry. Effect is not as noticeable on this hair type as it is with the curlier hair types (i.e. coiled and kinky). What this means is that most of the hairstyles you see done on straight hair can be done on your mane if you happen to have wavy hair. Pomade, hair gel, hair mousse and wax (use wax only at short and medium lengths) are your best products to use; the leave-in conditioner is used as a hairstyling foundation (i.e. applied first), and it starts to become a necessity at medium lengths.

- The Caesar Cut (short length)

This is a short-length hairstyle that involves having your back and sides of the head cropped with a hair clipper (preferably done as a taper) while leaving the top trimmed evenly with any length between 0.5 to 1 inches. You style the hair on the top of your head in a forward direction, starting from the crown area and ending at the forehead's hairline as you leave a short vertical fringe laying on the forehead. Use a wide-tooth comb to style the hair forward and your fingers to further style the short fringe.

An awesome-mane example of the Caesar Cut is that of George Clooney in the 1996 movie From Dusk Till Dawn.

- The Metro Mullet (short length)

The Metro Mullet is a short-length mullet-like hairstyle that I originally coined after seeing this new hairstyle being sported by Cristiano Ronaldo. The Metro Mullet is quite an innovative hairstyle that I saw emulated by young men in Europe (especially in southern Europe) after Cristiano Ronaldo. Because the hairstyle had no actual name, I decided to popularise it online by calling it the "Metro Mullet" ("Metro" indicating that it is an urban and stylised version of a mullet).

The Metro Mullet has the scalp with 3 different hair lengths: the sides of the head are cropped at a #2 and tapered, the top of the head is kept at an even length of 1-2 inches, and then the back of the head is tapered down (starting at the vertex) with scissors until 1 inch before the nape's hairline. The hair located on the area of the back of the head encompassing 1 inch above the nape's hairline all the way down to the nape itself is to be the same length as the hair on the top of the head; thus, a pseudo mullet is created as the hair on the back of the head gradually decreases in length and then promptly increases in length again just above the nape. Another version of the Metro Mullet (albeit less stylised) is performed by leaving the hair on the back of the head at the same length as the hair on the top of the head (instead of having the hair tapered) and then having the mullet 1 inch longer than the hair on the top/back of the head.

The hair on the top and upper back of the head is to be styled in the same manner. The hair can be lifted up with the fingers (puffed out), can be parted to the side or can be directed towards the centre to create a crest (refer to the Faux Hawk hairstyle for coiled hair). The Mullet is flared out with your fingers to make it a bit more visible, and you can also spike it or puff it out.

Cristiano Ronaldo sported a Metro Mullet during the 2006 FIFA World Cup, and he has been spotted with this hairstyle on and off ever since.

- The Side Swept (medium length)

This is a medium-length hairstyle in which you have your sides and back trimmed up to 1 inch while leaving the top between 2-4 inches. All the hair on the top is parted (swept) to one side, and the line of division for the part is drawn starting at either the left or right temple of your head. Unlike the Side Fringe hairstyle, which also shares the side parting at the temple, there is no fringe here: all of the hair on the top of the head is parted to the side so that the newly-swept hair remains perpendicular or at an angle to the parted line created.

A dude who wears the Side Swept with style and class is Billy Zane in the movie Titanic.

- The Undercut (medium length)

This hairstyle involves having your back and sides cropped to an even #2 while the top is left anywhere from 2-4 inches even. The hair on the top is then slicked either back or to the side, and you can either leave the hair to puff out a bit or have it flattened. If you choose to have some volume on the hair, use hair mousse and a hair drier, and then finish off by using a bit of pomade to coat your waves as you continue to lift the hair up. On the other hand, if you choose to have a flatter top, use either wax or pomade to slick the hair back or to the side. Use a wide-tooth comb for the manipulation of the hairstyle.

German soccer player Mario Gomez, who plays for Bayern Munich, is fond of the Undercut hairstyle and sported it during the UEFA Euro 2012 tournament.

- The Jim Morrison (long length)

The Jim Morrison is a hairstyle named after the rock star himself, Jim Morrison. To achieve this hairstyle, you need 6 inches of hair all around your head. To style a Jim Morrison, use hair mousse to lift your hair up so that it ends up looking like a helmet. Use your fingers to lift the hair up, aiming to create a visual helmet-like effect. If you use a leave-in conditioner normally as your hairstyling foundation, it is best that for this particular hairstyle you either use a smaller-than-usual amount or skip the leave-in altogether to style your mane in a Jim Morrison because the leave-in will weight down your waves. While the Jim Morrison is not a fully puffing-out hairstyle, it certainly requires a messy volume that defies gravity somewhat.

With the Jim Morrison hairstyle, you want to elongate the lifting-up motion of your fingers and solely use hair mousse as a hairstyling agent so that the waves can defy gravity. You can also use a hair dryer to enhance the puffing out of the hair.

Jim Morrison in any of the covers for The Best Of albums of The Doors will serve to illustrate this wild hairstyle.

## Coiled hair

Coiled hair will have a tendency to defy gravity until it reaches at least 8 inches in visible length, and it will puff out when shorter. Because this hair type is formed as coils rather than waves, you want to use plenty of leave-in conditioner and avoid sweeping or excessively slicking your hair. The Damp vs. Dry effect is noticeable with coiled hair so watch out for it: your hair will not look the same when it dries as it did when it was damp and styled! Use a leave-in conditioner at all times, either as a standalone hairstyling agent or as a foundation to other agents; you can also use hair gel, hair mousse, pomade, styling creams and hair spray. Avoid hair wax except for short-length coils and only use it in small amounts.

- The Crew Cut (short length)

This hairstyle is great for short-length coiled hair as it is convenient and can be customised as per one's taste. The top is cropped very short and tapered from the crown towards the front so that the front has a little bit more length than the crown. The sides and back are kept even shorter, from a #1 to a #2, and done in a taper too. This hairstyle is similar to the High and Tight (recommended for kinky hair), only that the length differences between the top, sides and back of the head are much smaller and less noticeable in the Crew Cut hairstyle. Another cool thing of this hairstyle is that you can customise it with lines and even patches of shaved hair, making elaborate designs as the length of the hairstyle itself is very short anyway, which allows for creative dents in the hair (I recommend you to have the barber do it, not do it yourself).

A great example of how good a Crew Cut hairstyle can look on a curly male is the hair of United State's President Barack Obama in his earlier political career as a senator.

- The Faux Hawk (short length)

This hairstyle is a trendy one with young urban males. It revolves around styling the hair on the top of the head towards the middle so as to form a crest running from the centre of the forehead's hairline to the crown area. You will need your sides and back tapered to a #2 with a hair clipper, and the top should be anywhere from 0.5 to 2 inches in height (i.e. visible length). The Faux Hawk is a modern alternative to the extreme Mohawk hairstyle and suits short coils greatly. Use your fingers to define the crest and use either your fingers or a wide-tooth comb to direct the hair on the top of the head towards the middle so as to form the crest. The crest can be as wide as you want it to be although 0.5-inches wide all across the crest is a good width to shoot for.

A great example of the Faux Hawk hairstyle is that of Cristiano Ronaldo playing for Real Madrid in the 2010-2011 Spanish soccer league.

- The Jewfro (medium length)

The Jewfro is a popular hairstyle for coiled-haired men. The name itself comes from the popularity of this hairstyle among males of Jewish heritage, for whom coiled hair is a common trait. It is similar in goal to the common Afro hairstyle in that the hair is allowed to puff out and look voluminous. You will need the same length all around your head (preferably 3-5 inches), and you will use hair mousse to lift the hair up when it is damp. Run your fingers coated with hair mousse from mid-length to the tips so that the whole length gets coated with hair mousse, and emphasise the lifting up and puffing out of your coils.

The good thing about hair mousse is that it is easy to remove and hardly leaves any residue, so it is OK if some hair mousse unintentionally coats the base of the hair strands when you are styling your Jewfro. Moreover, while the Jewfro and the Jim Morrison hairstyles share a puffing-out emphasis, you should use some leave-in conditioner for the Jewfro as a foundation prior to applying the hair mousse. You can blow-dry the Jewfro too, but don't go overboard and do leave some dampness in the hair.

Many coiled-haired men make the mistake of allowing their hair to become dry and frizzy, which then leads to their curly hair naturally taking the form of a pseudo Jewfro. The thing is, you are reading this book because you want great-looking hair, not a frizzy dead rat on top of your head; hence, the Jewfro should not be the result of allowing your curls to become dry but the result of having a mane that is moisturised and styled accordingly and which looks awesome regardless of the hairstyle. I grow quite the Jewfro myself, and I can tell you that the difference between a dry Jewfro and a moisturised Jewfro is like day and night (not to mention that women love an awesome Jewfro mane as it really flaunts your coils).

An example of a male with an awesome Jewfro is Justin Guarini, a popular American singer who has sported this hairstyle for most of his career since 2002.

- The Hanging Locks (long length)

The Hanging Locks hairstyle is perfect for long coiled hair because it doesn't take a huge amount of time for this hair type to hang down (as opposed to kinky hair), and the hanging down can be enhanced with the use of hairstyling agents that add weight to the hair strands. With the Hanging Locks hairstyle, you will need 10 inches of extended hair length on the top, and the sides and back should be 8 inches, which will give a very full appearance to your mane.

For the Hanging Locks hairstyle, I recommend you to use a styling cream so as to ensure that the locks hang down, for, at the aforementioned stipulated lengths, coiled hair tends not to hang down fully without hair products. Coat your coils with leave-in conditioner first, then add the styling cream. Once the hair is coated with these 2 hairstyling agents, shake your coils and let them hang down freely without parting them to the side. Slick back any locks hanging on your face but don't manipulate the rest of the hair.

A perfect male example of this hairstyle is David Bisbal in the cover of his 2004 album Buleria.

- The Beyond Shoulder Length (long length)

This hairstyle requires you to grow your coiled hair beyond shoulder length (so much longer than the Hanging Locks hairstyle). A good length to aim for is chest length because at this length your locks will be hanging down without the need of hair products while expressing great follicular volume: a true lion's mane! If you are growing from a short length, this hairstyle will take you about 5 years to achieve, but it is a great hairstyle if you want to really sport an impressive head of Es. What's more is that since you will be growing your coils already with an optimised hair-care and hair-grooming approach, your hair will be looking great throughout the entire journey that it takes you to have your hair reaching its final length.

For the Beyond Shoulder Length hairstyle, it is best that you grow your mane starting from an even length all around your head. Moreover, you should not go for trims until you achieve the final length desired (only go for trims if you have damaged the tips of the hair). It is imperative to keep your hair free of tangles with this hairstyle as you can get some vicious knots and tangles appearing very fast, so use a leave-in conditioner every day and a normal conditioner on just about all days too.

NFL player Troy Polamalu of the Pittsburgh Steelers is the perfect example of what coiled hair grown beyond shoulder length can look like.

## Kinky hair

Kinky hair can vary between a blend of tightly-formed Es and Zs to a head full of Zs, thus this hair type thrives best when not manipulated. If you are the proud owner of kinky hair, do not try to sweep it or dominate it with hairstyles. Kinky hair is a step up from coiled hair in terms of volume, and your best approach is to embrace the natural volume yielded by your particular curls, hence it is with kinky hair that the Shake & Go hairstyle is of greatest use. The Damp vs. Dry effect is very noticeable once the kinks reach a medium length; thus, you should not try to fight your hair and instead embrace its voluminous nature.

A leave-in conditioner is a must, and natural oils and butters are great add-ons for your styling stage. Hair gels, pomades and styling creams are also great options though try to emphasise the use of a leave-in conditioner as the foundation for your styling and then add the rest of your chosen hairstyling agents, paying particular attention to not getting any of them on your scalp.

- The High and Tight (short length)

The High and Tight is a great hairstyle for those with kinky hair who want to sport a low-maintenance, good-looking hairstyle. With the High and Tight, you will crop the back and sides of your scalp to a #2 while the top is left anywhere from a #4 to a trimmed length of up to 1 inch. You can go lower than a #2 with the guard length for the sides and back, but do a #2 first, then leave 2-3 weeks before you crop the hair shorter to make sure that your scalp gets tanned naturally to the same tone as your face, otherwise you will have a disturbing skin tone discrepancy between your face and the sides and back of your head. The top of your head can either be styled with your fingers or styled with a wide-tooth comb.

A great example of a High and Tight is that of Shemar Moore in the TV show Criminal Minds.

- The Shake & Go (medium length)

Because kinky hair thrives with the least manipulation, the Shake & Go hairstyle is perfect to flaunt those kinks of yours. Get your hair to an even medium length (preferably 4-5 inches) all around your head; to style, simply coat your damp Zs with a leave-in conditioner and your other chosen hairstyling agents, then shake your head, and you are ready to go. Since your hair will already be optimised via your hair grooming, your kinks will be allowed to express themselves while looking great as you will have developed the habits needed to have a great-looking mane. For the Shake & Go hairstyle, you can finish off the styling stage by adding a fingertip amount of coconut butter or any other natural oil or butter to the tip of your locks for an extra hair-conditioning layer.

The Shake & Go is very similar in concept to the Hanging Locks hairstyle for long coiled hair, only that, with the Shake & Go hairstyle as done on medium-length kinks, your hair will not hang down and will instead defy gravity.

Corbin Bleu, in the TV movie High School Musical, is a great male illustration of the Shake & Go hairstyle.

- The Afro (medium length)

This hairstyle is the everest of mane awesomeness for kinky-haired dudes. If your curls are of the kinky type, the Afro hairstyle is a great way to acknowledge your mane, and this hairstyle always looks great when it is taken care of. Most commonly a medium-length hairstyle, your Afro should have an even length all around your head, with the chosen even length for your kinks being anywhere from 2 to 6 inches. It is imperative for you to keep your Afro moisturised daily with plenty of leave-in conditioner and by coating the tips with natural oils and butters because the main problem with not achieving mane awesomeness with the Afro hairstyle is failing to keep the kinks moisturised.

The Afro hairstyle is greatly illustrated by Lenny Kravitz any time that he is not sporting dreadlocks or a Buzz Cut (he seems to prefer the Afro for his medium-length hairstyle).

- Braids (long length)

Braids are a favourite for men with long kinky hair. Due to the tightness of the kinks, this hair type has a tendency to defy gravity even at very long lengths. Instead, braids pair up the long Z-shaped locks, allowing them to be weighted down and thus hang down. A good way to approach the braided hairstyle is to transition from an Afro to braids: once your Afro reaches a good-enough long length that you are happy with (e.g. 10 inches), then braid your mane. It should be noted, however, that the braiding process and braids themselves put a lot of tension on the hair follicles, and this hairstyle can cause some unneeded hair loss if the hair is braided too tight, so you certainly want to use someone who knows how to braid hair if you decide to have your kinky mane braided.

Rapper Snoop Dogg is an awesome male example of how to rock braids as a kinky-haired male.

## Taking into account your Curl Factor for your hairstyles

As you know, your Curl Factor will have a direct influence in the difference between how your hair looks when you style it and how your hair looks when it fully dries (i.e. the Damp vs. Dry effect). The coiled and kinky hair types have the highest Curl Factor, which means that you should be striving to manipulate your hair the least if you have any of these 2 hair types.

To slightly influence the Curl Factor (i.e. have it lowered), you goal is to retain as much extended length as possible when the hair starts to dry. Thus, you should use hairstyling agents that add significant weight to the hair strands: strong-hold hair gels, styling creams and leave-in conditioners are your best allies for this goal.

To influence the Damp vs. Dry effect, you should avoid hairstyles that have you sweeping or parting your hair excessively; this being the reason why I haven't included any heavy-duty sweeping hairstyles on my list of recommended hairstyles for coiled and kinky hair. If you want to ensure that your hairstyle remains the same as it dries, you have 2 options:

1. Go with the Shake & Go hairstyle or a variation thereof in which the hair is not swept nor parted (except for any removing of locks hanging on your face).

2. Use a blow dryer to remove some of the dampness off the hair, aiming to leave the hair still somewhat damp and using your fingers to style the hair.

These 2 options listed work best for the coiled and kinky hair types, but they too work for straight and wavy hair despite the Damp vs. Dry effect not being as prominent in the latter 2 hair types.

# Straightening your hair

You may not always want to sport the same hairstyles over and over or have the same hair type, so straightening your hair opens a new door to the hairstyles that you can sport at any given time. This hair-modifying method is most commonly done to have one's hair changed from any of the curly hair types to the straight hair type. However, one can simply loosen up his curls instead of having them fully straightened; an example of this would be loosening up the curls from kinky to wavy.

There are 2 methods to straighten your hair: using a straightening iron and using a straightening product. Both methods work to alter the structure of the hair although one is temporary (straightening iron) whereas the other is permanent (straightening product). The main problem with either of these 2 straightening methods is that each time you use them, you create small amounts of damage in the hair shafts, which means that, if you want to go back to your normal hair type, your hair will not look as great as it did before straightening it. Thus, I encourage you to work within your hair type and only straighten your hair after having given it a good thought; many guys who have come to me in the past for advice on their fried-looking hair have told me that they weren't aware of how straightening their hair could negatively affect their natural hair type so much and that they would have straightened their hair much more conservatively had they known this fact beforehand.

## Using a straightening iron

Also known as a flat iron or hair straightener, a straightening iron is a device that temporarily straightens the hair by heating it and altering its structure. The iron itself is in the form of 2 plates that open up and then close to provide heat, and you put a lock or a bunch of locks from your mane in between the opened, heated plates, then closing the plates and running the iron along the entire length of the plate-clipped lock/s. The straightening result is instant, but your hair will return to its original hair type when you wet it again.

Improper use of a straightening iron can literally fry your hair as will straightening your hair day in and day out. To minimise damage to your hair when using a straightening iron, make sure that you first apply a heat protectant (i.e. heat-protecting product) and use the lowest temperature available in the settings of the iron. Likewise, try to only use the straightening iron occasionally (e.g on certain days you want to rock a different look). Lastly, up your normal conditioner frequency to the "50% off days" rule if you will be straightening your hair with the iron more than once a week.

If you have straight hair, you can still use a straightening iron to add definition to a hairstyle (i.e. straightening the fringe on your forehead).

## Using a straightening product

Straightening products are known as hair relaxers and are products that are meant to be left on the hair for a certain amount of time (20+ minutes) so as to fully straighten the hair. Relaxers contain chemicals that alter the structure of the hair, rendering the hair straight. The results are permanent, but are only so for the hair that has been "relaxed" (i.e. had the relaxer applied to); the hair that is to grow after the relaxer will grow back in your usual hair type.

There are other straightening products which do not fully straighten the hair and instead loosen up the curls; these products are known as texturisers and are left on your hair for a shorter amount of time than relaxers. Texturisers are most commonly used with kinky hair to loosen up the curl and allow for easier management of the curls.

For best results, it is best to go to the hairdresser to get your hair relaxed or texturised, at least for the first time you decide to try one of these products. Both relaxers and texturisers require some special manipulation as well as strict following of the instructions; otherwise, you run the risk of not only excessively damaging your hair but also burning your scalp.

If you relax or texturise your hair, up your normal conditioning frequency in the same manner as if you were using a straightening iron (i.e. the "50% off days" rule). Because the results are permanent with relaxers/texturisers, your hair will be more prone to breaking off, which means that you should avoid any excessive manipulation of your hair; only use your fingers to style your hair and do not tie your hair tightly.

## How to choose the right barber

Many times, we males underestimate the benefit of having a good barber or hairdresser. Indeed, to be able to rock the best-looking hair that you possibly can, you also need to be in the hands of a good hair professional. Not all barbers and hairdressers are created equal, and you want to choose one who has experience with your hair type and who is also a good listener.

How many times have you stepped inside a barbershop or hair salon to get a haircut and left with something completely different to what you wanted? How many times did you trust the barber to do what he felt was right, only to find that what he thought was right differed vastly from what you thought was right? If you are like me, your experiences with barbers and hairdressers are more on the bad side than on the good side, and you try to avoid them unless necessary.

Having a great-looking mane relies on you doing everything right, but, when the time comes for a good haircut (and it will come), you can either do it yourself or have someone else doing it for you. And while I am one who thinks that for things to go your way, you need to be the one doing them; a good haircut is best relied on a hair professional. By all means, have a go at cutting your own hair and learn how to give yourself frequent trims, but I recommend you to go to a barber or hairdresser whenever you need a good haircut.

Once you start putting all your acquired hair knowledge into practice, you will learn to appreciate your hair, and your first time stepping inside a barber or hair salon with your finally-optimised mane will give you butterflies in the stomach. Due to your newly-found appreciation for your hair, you will not be very receptive to someone else touching and manipulating your hair, so you must know how to choose the right professional for your haircut. I have walked out of a barbershop after being there for 5 minutes and seeing the guy who went before me getting a horrible haircut by a hairdresser who thought a "hip" haircut consisted of leaving lumps of hair on each side of the head while buzzing the top. The guy getting the haircut didn't look like he was enjoying having the hairdresser (or "hairkiller" as it looked) freestyling a haircut on his head, and I was pretty much terrified of having that hairdresser dude within 10 feet of my head.

To ensure choosing the best barber or hairdresser right from the very beginning and getting the most out of him/her, follow these points:

- Be 100% sure of what haircut you want. Practise describing what haircut you want to a friend or family member: if they can understand what you want done, a hair professional will have no problems catching your 100% drift.

- Take pictures with you to the barber. Take magazines, printed pictures, newspaper clippings or whatever illustrations needed to show him what it is that you want done.

- A good barber/hairdresser should know how to cut hair when dry. Curly hair, be it wavy, coiled or kinky, should be cut dry most of the time because, if it is cut when wet or damp, it is difficult to assess how the haircut will look when the hair dries due to the Damp vs. Dry effect. Ask him if he is familiarised with cutting hair dry if you have curly hair.

- Be realistic, not all haircuts will suit you. While George Clooney may look awesome with a Caesar Cut, you may not fare just as well because you don't have his facial structure. Ideally, you want to have 3 haircuts in mind and discuss with the barber which one of the 3 would suit you best. Barbers and hairdressers have seen and worked on all sort of faces and hair, so they will be able to advise you on how each haircut will suit you.

- Remember, a good barber/hairdresser always listens to you. You should spend about 5 minutes in the beginning talking about what you want done, and you should be asking him for his opinion, feedback, and any alternatives he has to what you have proposed. Don't worry about being overly detailed and spend as much time as needed to make sure that you both are on the same page. It only takes him 2 seconds to chop by mistake 1 inch from a hair lock of yours, yet it will take you at least 2 months to grow back that lost hair length. Go out of your way to be as precise and detailed as possible so that he/she can then deliver a good job; that way, if the hairdresser provides a good-enough service,

*(follows from previous page)*

you can then become a regular and he/she will know your particular case and give you a more-customised service.

- Be aware at all times that a haircut is different from a hairstyle, and sometimes even barbers get themselves confused with these 2 terms. A haircut can be done in minutes, but a hairstyle will require you to style your hair day in and day out. Are you sure you want to get a specific haircut that only allows you to style your hair in a particular hairstyle every day for the next 2 months? If you want to be flexible with hairstyles, choose a haircut that will allow you to choose from several hairstyles in any given day and that will not limit you to just one.

- For us dudes, barbers tend to be a better option than hairdressers when it comes to convenience. Barbers are used to cutting hair for males who want good hair but also want convenient hair. Hairdressers (and hairstylists), on the other hand, tend to be experienced in giving haircuts that look good in the given moment but are a pain in the derriere to style every day. Overall, I find barbers to be more suited for men's haircuts than hairdressers, but there are some pretty good hairdressers out there too. Research him/her fully before making your decision, and do not hesitate to visit him and have a chat with him or his assistants before making a decision.

- Try to find a barber/hairdresser who has plenty of experience with curly hair and especially with your hair type. Curly hair is different to cut than straight hair, and there are bits and pieces that a barber/hairdresser needs to master to be able to provide a good haircut to a curly-haired male. Even if you have straight hair, choosing a barber who knows how to properly cut curly hair guarantees yourself a barber who takes the time to study and learn, not just chop hair generically. Ask him how much experience he has with curly hair and with your specific hair type.

- Female barbers/hairdressers are just as capable as males in delivering a great haircut. The only thing different is that a male barber will be obviously more aware of your needs as a man. All other things equal, I normally go for a male

*(follows from previous page)*

barber because I know that I can relate to him in terms of sporting a masculine haircut. Likewise, it totally kills my mood to have to be waiting my turn in a hair salon full of old women with foil covering their hair and reading the latest issue of Cosmopolitan. Horses for courses though, and, as I say, both genders are equally capable of delivering a great haircut and service.

- Don't go by price. My best haircut was done in Alabama by a barber who charged me $6. My worst haircut was one I had in London by a hairdresser who charged me $35 for a fade and scissor-trimmed top (I was new in the city and desperate for a haircut). Actually, let me take that back: my best haircut ever was when I was 21 and my friends and I were at a house party doing tequila contests. I beat one of my friends, so I, in a drunken stupor, asked him to cut my hair in front of everyone in the house. He was even more drunk than I was and had his right hand in a sling, yet he miraculously got to performing on my scalp an awesome High and Tight that looked out of this world. We are talking about cutting hair here, not performing brain surgery, so there's no need to break the bank to get a great and convenient haircut.

- Arrive at the hair salon some 15 minutes before scheduled so that you can see how your chosen hair professional performs his job with someone else (why be the guinea pig when you can have someone else be experimented on?). See how much attention the barber/hairdresser pays to what he is doing and if he is detailed enough. Try to hear if he chats while performing the haircut. I recommend you to never choose a barber/hairdresser who doesn't look like he is paying much attention to the haircut or talks too much while doing his job. While I understand that a barber or a hairdresser might have to be on his feet cutting hair for 10+ hours, it is a reality that one cannot do 2 things perfectly at the same time. Moreover, if he is doing all the talking, it means he is not doing the listening (to you).

- Do not be afraid to walk out of the barbershop/hair salon if you are not 100% sure of the hairdresser's ability to deliver a professional service. You would not be the first one to walk out on a hairdresser, and you would not be the last one either. Remember, you now have an optimised mane, not a dead rat that can be abused and cut like a rag. Be aware though that you may still be liable for paying the unperformed service, especially if you made an appointment.

- Lastly, build a relationship with your barber or hairdresser. This is because you want him to know your hair and your circumstances, which will allow him to offer you the best service possible. Strive to find someone who fits the profile shaped by the list of points you have just read: good listener, professional and has experience with your hair type. Once you find him or her, do not let him go because a good barber/hairdresser is hard to find for a second time!

## Hair accessories to enhance your locks

Men have used hair accessories for centuries, either as ornaments for their manes to showcase their social status or as tools to keep their hair fixed when engaging in battle or physical activity. The popularity of hair accessories faded as shorter hairstyles became more popular at the turn of the 20th century, but hair accessories have made a comeback in the last decade as urban men have started to enhance their image in the most creative of manners.

The following are the hair accessories that I recommend for your hair:

- Headbands

- Hair bands

- Bobby pins

- Do-rags

- Hair picks

The above 5 hair accessories serve a tangible purpose while blending in nicely with your male hair, and they are the ones that I recommend if you want to enhance your Is, Ss, Es or Zs.

I will not deny it; the correct use of hair accessories is a bit tricky for us men. You must choose them wisely as it is very easy to ruin an already-aesthetic mane; thus, when in doubt, do not wear hair accessories. You should bear in mind the following when deciding to wear any hair accessory:

- Discretion: the hair accessory is there to enhance your mane, not to take away from it. Never wear a hair accessory just because you want to show off your latest acquisition. Remember, your hair is already looking great through its proper grooming and caring, so do not detract from it with silly hair accessories.

- Choose the appropriate colour: always choose a hair accessory that resembles the colour of your hair. So, if you have black hair, go for black or dark-brown accessories. Blue or green-coloured hair accessories are out of the hair equation (although you can use grey-coloured ones if you want).

- Go for cotton or cloth-made hair accessories whenever possible: this means avoid using rubber bands from the office and don't get hair bands that have metallic bits. Cotton and cloth-made hair accessories are gentle on the hair and won't damage your awesome mane, so always choose textile-based ones.

- Consider the length of your hair: most hair accessories are best used when your hair has reached at least a medium length. Stay away from wearing hair accessories when your hair is short as most hair accessories don't serve a tangible purpose for this hair-length category (except do-rags).

The aforementioned 4 points should be the defining factors to consider when selecting the right hair accessory. Abide by them and remember: when in doubt, don't wear hair accessories!

These are the details of the specific hair accessories that I recommend:

## Headbands

These are bands that are wrapped around your head to pull the hair back. They are ideal for those times when you are doing some form of physical activity and need to have a clear visual field (i.e. your hair doesn't block your eyesight). Headbands are very popular among male sportsmen such as soccer and tennis players, and headbands can be used in social settings too.

Use headbands when your hair is at least a medium length. Stick to headbands made of cotton or other textile material and choose those that are no wider than an inch. Stay away from plastic headbands and blend the colour of the headband with your natural hair colour.

## Hair bands

Also known as hair ties, hair bands are the smaller version of headbands, and they are used to tie the hair into a ponytail, braid or bun. They are very useful to secure the hair when you need the most assurance that your hair won't be moving around. Hair bands also work great for when the occasion calls for a neat look with long hair (e.g. in the workplace).

Hair bands should be used when your hair is at a medium or long length and can be tied. Again, choose the hair band according to the colour of your hair, and avoid hair bands that have metallic bits in them.

## Bobby pins

These are discreet and thin metallic pins that are useful for securing your hair in place without making it look like you have anything in your hair. They are best used when your hair is at a long length, and you should only use a few at a time. Bobby pins take some skill to master, and I recommend you to ask any females whom you know about how to use bobby pins since most ladies use them or know how to use them. Bobby pins are not difficult to use, for you only have to clip them to any locks you want to have held in position, but you need to practise with bobby pins to have them working efficiently. It is imperative that you choose bobby pins that match your hair colour as they should not be visible at first sight.

## Do-rags

The do-rag is a fitting piece of cloth that is used to cover the scalp and is useful for preserving your locks from daily wear and tear as well as for any instances where you will be rubbing your hair against anything (including on a windy day). The bandana is similar to the do-rag, only that the former tends to be less fitting around the head than the latter.

Unlike the previous hair accessories, do-rags can be used with any hair length, including near-shaved.

## Hair picks

Also known as afro picks, hair picks should be used mostly by those with an Afro hairstyle (kinky hair). This is because the great volume of the Afro hairstyle in kinky hair allows for the hair pick to be held in place; no other hairstyle or hair type can hold a hair pick in place like the Afro hairstyle in this curliest of hair types hence the hair pick's specific use. The hair pick is very useful to retouch one's Afro and detangle any formed knots, and it has become a fashionable item to sport on one's mane provided that the hair is such hair type and in such hairstyle.

# Growing hair long

More and more males are venturing into growing their hair beyond short and medium lengths. Long hair in males can look great provided that it is looked after properly; thus, because you now know how to optimally look after your hair and implement its grooming, growing your hair long becomes are very real possibility that you can now consider.

As you've learnt, hair grows 0.5 inches of extended length, which means that straight hair will achieve a visible length faster than the curly hair types; this being one of the reasons why the vast majority of men with long hair have straight hair; it just takes too long for the curly hair types to manifest their visible length! Wavy, coiled and kinky hair will bend and curve along the way, limiting their ability to display the longest (visible) length. However, regardless of your hair type, you can indeed grow your hair long and have it looking great.

In Chapter 2, you learnt about the Curl Factor, and it is precisely this hair-profiling element that influences your ability to reach certain visible lengths. A classic example illustrating the Curl Factor discrepancy between straight hair and kinky hair is when someone with kinky hair straightens his hair (e.g. with a straightening iron) and suddenly sees how long his hair actually is. Same with when you are showering, if you hair is a medium length or longer, you will have noticed that your hair reaches your eyes (and beyond) when the hair is soaked, yet the hair looks much shorter when it dries fully as it curls back into its natural state.

Since the Curl Factor is a novel concept that I have created in the hair-care industry, I have experimented with my hair and the hair of others to see how it influenced the ability of one to grow his hair to certain visible and extended lengths. For example, a typical distance between the top of your head and the base of the neck is 12 inches (give or take some inches depending on your height and how you measure the distance); ergo, someone with straight hair will only take 24 months to have all of his hair reach the base of his neck (at 0.5 inches of extended length per month) whereas someone with wavy, coiled or kinky hair will take much longer because his hair will be taking the longest distance (i.e. bend and curve) to reach the base of the neck. Mind, you both males are growing the same 0.5 inches of extended hair length per month, but the wavy, coiled or kinky-haired male is obviously not getting the full 0.5 inches as visible length.

<u>Figure 22 – A straight line (i.e. non-curly hair) and a non-straight line (i.e. curly hair)</u>

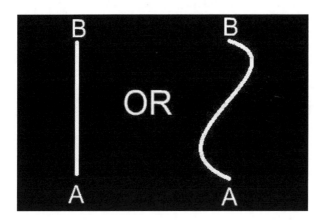

The above is why curly men complain about never being able to grow their hair long. It can literally take a male with curly hair (i.e. kinky) 3 times longer to have his hair reach a certain body part (e.g. shoulder or ears) than a straight-haired male. And that's not counting the notorious issue of the hair puffing out with coiled and kinky hair.

So as to give you the most bang for your buck, I have created the next table (Figure 23) that outlines how long (in months) it will take for your hair type to reach certain visible lengths (2, 4, 6, 12 inches) starting from a shaved length (0 inches).

Figure 23 – Timespan in months growing from a shaved length (0 inches) to stipulated visible lengths

|  | Shaved | 2 inches | 4 inches | 6 inches | 12 inches |
|---|---|---|---|---|---|
| Straight | 0 | 4 | 8 | 12 | 24 |
| Wavy | 0 | 6 | 12 | 18 | 36 |
| Coiled | 0 | 10 | 20 | 30 | 60 |
| Kinky | 0 | 12 | 24 | 36 | 72 |

Remember, the table above illustrates the months that it will take for your hair to grow to those visible lengths if you start growing your hair from a shaved length. Now, if your current visible length is not 0 (i.e. shaved), then round down your current visible length to any of the visible lengths accounted for in the table (2, 4, 6, or 12 inches); use the stated number of months for your rounded visible length and subtract that number from the number of months for your desired new visible length. Always round down your visible length, not round up (e.g. if your visible length is 3 inches, then use the number of months for the 2-inch column in the table, not the 4-inch column).

For example, let's say you have 5 inches of visible length for your coiled hair and you want to grow your curls to 12 inches. What you'd then do is subtract the number of months for your current length (20 months, 4-inch column) from the number of months for your desired new length (60 months, 12-inch column). Thus, it'd take you 40 months (60 minus 20) to have your coiled hair at your current length reaching a visible length of 12 inches. Or, in other words, it'd take you 40 months (almost 3.5 years) to have your locks touching your shoulders (i.e. base of the neck) if you start growing your hair now.

The number of months for each visible length in the table are estimations. They are numbers that have come from my years of researching and testing my concepts on the hair of others. Hence, you may find that you take a bit less (or more) time than forecasted with the table: some men happen to grow less/more than 0.5 inches of extended length per month, and your hair growth rate can easily be affected by your nutrition. In fact, you will probably find that your hair grows not only healthier but also faster once you optimise your nutrition as per your hair-care aspect. In any case, it is always better to be conservative with hair-growth forecasts, and always plan for the longest scenario. Going back to the coiled-hair example on the previous paragraph, you'd known that, at the very least, you should expect 40 months (not any less) to have your hair reaching 12 inches of visible length.

Following from the above, I have also created a useful table (Figure 24) that will give you an approximation of your extended length at whichever visible length it is (and viceversa). This table illustrates how much hair you really need to grow if you have any of the curly hair types, for the difference between extended and visible length with the 3 curly hair types is quite noticeable.

Figure 24 – Equivalent of extended lengths (inches) at stipulated visible lengths

| | Shaved | 2 inches | 4 inches | 6 inches | 12 inches |
|---|---|---|---|---|---|
| Straight | 0 | 2 | 4 | 6 | 12 |
| Wavy | 0 | 3 | 6 | 9 | 18 |
| Coiled | 0 | 5 | 10 | 15 | 30 |
| Kinky | 0 | 6 | 12 | 18 | 36 |

Growing your hair long (6+ inches) will require more hair-management efforts from your part, albeit the structure and system of the hair-management equation is the same. The only thing changing is that, since you will have more hair mass, you will take a bit longer to do your daily hair grooming. Likewise, you will find that you have to implement more hair-care measures than when your hair was shorter (e.g. you will have to tie your hair when it is windy).

Like I say, your hair-management efforts will be a bit more intensive when your hair is long, but, so long as you abide by your hair-management equation, your long-hair efforts will not impair your lifestyle and will be on auto-pilot. Furthermore, don't worry about your hair growth per se and instead worry about supplying your follicles with the right nutrients for optimal hair growth.

# Conclusion

Your mane will be shaped by your hairstyle and any accessories you may so choose to use. Regardless of your hair type and hair length, you have hairstyles available to you, and you must always be realistic about what can and can't be done with your hair in terms of styles. Your Curl Factor and Damp vs. Dry effect will be decisive in the types of hairstyles that you can use, and you can influence these 2 hair-profiling elements somewhat. However, it's in your interest to roll with your unique hair (including its type) instead of trying to adapt your hair to hairstyles that are just too elaborate or complex for your particular hair type, hair length, Curl Factor or Damp vs. Dry effect.

Straightening your hair is a viable option if you have any of the curly hair types. You must understand though that, every time you straighten your hair, you create some damage to your hair, which will cause your hair to not look 100% as it used to before you started straightening it. The good thing though about straightening your hair is that it opens a whole new door of hairstyles for you, and you can always outgrow the hair that is minimally-damaged from the straightening.

So far, you have learnt all about how you should optimise your hair-management equation by yourself. Nevertheless, the time will come when you have to rely on others (i.e. hair professionals) to help you achieve the best-looking mane possible. Thus, you must know how to shop around for a good hair professional, and you want to establish a relationship with your chosen barber or hairdresser so that he/she knows your hair fully and can then offer you the best service possible.

Growing your hair long will take more or less time depending on your hair type and, by default, on your Curl Factor too. Visible length is what matters when it comes to having your hair reach a certain body part, so you should be using the tables given in this chapter to work out how long it will take you to grow your hair. Furthermore, hair that is long (6+ inches) will carry the most effort-investing management (compared to hair at short and medium lengths), but having long hair is definitively possible as a modern male so long as you abide by your hair-management equation.

# Anthony's barbershop case study

Patel was an 18-year old straight-haired male who had just started college. He had come to Anthony because he (Patel) wanted to change his hair's look. Until then, Patel had sported a neat Ivy League-like hairstyle as imposed from his conservative parents, but, now that he was on his own at college and partying every week, Patel wanted to have a cooler, more modern hairstyle.

Patel wasn't really sure what he wanted as a hairstyle; he simply asked Anthony to give him a cool hairstyle. Patel had very dense straight hair, so pretty much anything could be done on his hair. Anthony cropped Patel's sides and back, trimmed his hair a bit and gave Patel the instructions to give himself (Patel) the Shaggy hairstyle whenever he desired. Patel was very pleased with the results, and Anthony recommended Patel to, next time, come with specific hairstyles he had in mind. Anthony told Patel to bring any magazines or printed pictures of hairstyles that Patel would like to learn to give himself; that way, Anthony would be able to give Patel a more-customised look and service.

A month later, Patel came back to Anthony's barbershop for a trim and, this time, Patel brought a men's magazine that had a picture of Cristiano Ronaldo sporting a Faux Hawk and a picture of Mario Gomez sporting an Undercut (Patel loved soccer). Both hairstyles (Faux Hawk and Undercut) can be done on straight and wavy hair, and Anthony decided to give Patel the haircut and the hairstyling instructions for the Faux Hawk as Anthony knew that this hairstyle would suit Patel very much. Anthony gave Patel a haircut that enhanced the Faux Hawk and gave Patel the specific instructions to give himself the hairstyle every day (the same instructions that you've learnt in this chapter!). From there onwards, Patel learnt to use Anthony's experience to his advantage, and Patel would bring along specific pictures to the barbershop so as to get a more-customised service from Anthony.

# 7) Putting Everything Together: Go Out And Rock That Mane!

Identifying your hair type, measuring your 2 hair lengths, finding your optimal shampooing frequency, knowing what hairstyling agents to use, choosing a suitable hairstyle, knowing how to shop for a good barber; your eyes are probably dry from all the reading and digesting of information you've done so far in all these chapters. Not a problem; you are about to embark on a journey to mane awesomeness, and there's no need to rush it.

The goal now is to put some form of order in which to approach your journey so that you can get going and start taking actions to optimise your hair-management equation. Before putting all your newly-acquired hair knowledge into practice, however, you must be confident and positive about starting this peculiar journey. You must convince yourself at this stage that you now have everything in your power to get a great-looking head of Is, Ss, Es or Zs. So, if you weren't already positive about achieving such a follicular goal, then it's as simple as doing it right now: you are about to start a journey that will yield results very soon and that will improve your looks immensely as a modern male, and you have all the knowledge needed for it in this book. It doesn't get any easier than telling yourself that last sentence a couple of times to get immensely stoked about putting yourself to action with your hair!

The way that I have structured the preceding chapters is pretty much what the flow should be in terms of starting and continuing with your journey to better hair. This is the flow that I recommend for best results as it has you first profiling all that there is to your hair while building a wealth of knowledge that will then allow you to tackle the oh-so-important aspects of hair grooming and hair care.

Going with the recommended flow to set the path for your awesome mane, you must first familiarise yourself with all the hair-profiling content in Chapter 2 "Hair-Profiling Aspect: Get To Know Your Hair!" and start by putting into action the acquired knowledge in that chapter as the first step of your peculiar hair journey. What is to follow next is the chronological order of the steps and actions that I recommend you to implement and follow for your journey to mane awesomeness.

# Chronological order of the steps to take for your journey's actions

## Step 1: Know your hair type, hair lengths, length category, Curl Factor and Norwood stage

The whole of Chapter 2 deals with the profiling aspect of your hair-management equation; all the knowledge acquired in this chapter has you understanding your hair so that you can then associate and make sense of the actions taken with regards to your 2 remaining hair-management aspects: your hair grooming and hair care. Thus, you must have the following 4 elements worked out as the first step of your journey to optimise your hair-management equation: hair type, hair lengths (extended, visible and extended length category), Curl Factor and Norwood stage. Do also note down your hair ID as per the abbreviations of the hair-profiling elements.

If your current hair is damaged from having used chemicals or hair straighteners improperly, then get a haircut and start growing your hair from scratch, but this time do so applying the hair-equation system so as to grow great-looking, strong hair strands. Otherwise, use the reactive hair-care measure of scheduling a deep-conditioner session every 2 weeks on your shampooing day for the next 8 weeks. Be aware though that damaged hair will not respond as well as undamaged hair to your hair-management equation.

## Step 2: Get yourself the hair products

After working out all of the 4 elements in Step 1, move to your hair grooming. It is time to buy yourself (if you don't own already) a shampoo, a normal conditioner, a leave-in conditioner and a hairstyling agent. Use the tables in Appendix XXVII, Appendix XXVIII and Appendix XIX to work out which hairstyling agents suit your hair type and hair length. For the shampoo and conditioners, simply get conventional ones: a shampoo with a sulfate-type ingredient and the 2 conditioners with any of the ingredients listed in Question 7 of the Q&A chapter "Questions & Answers: The Miscellaneous Stuff You Will Ask Yourself". Don't make it overly complicated, your goal for now is to be as basic as it gets when it comes to hair-grooming products.

Also, throw away any hair brushes you may have, especially if you have any of the 3 curly hair types. From now on, your only hair-manipulating tools will be your fingers and a wide-tooth comb if you have curly hair (i.e. wavy, coiled or kinky) or your fingers and a conventional comb if you have straight hair (though you can also use a wide-tooth comb if you have straight hair). Purchase a wide-tooth comb that is either metallic or wooden, avoid plastic ones. You can buy at this stage a hair dryer and a hair straightener if you want, but you will not be using either of these 2 hair gadgets until you have your hair-grooming routine sorted out; you can also buy these 2 gadgets later on in your journey as they won't be of use just yet.

## Step 3: Know your natural hair for a week

Before finding your shampooing frequency and making use of your conditioning and hairstyling agents, you will go on a 7-day mission to know your natural hair. To start this hair-learning week, shampoo your hair the night before and then commence this special week the next morning; during the upcoming 7 days, you will not shampoo again, nor will you use anything else on your hair. Essentially, every day of this 7-day period will be a non-shampooing day, and you will only be performing the Sebum Coating method and your preferred hair-drying method, which will thus allow you to get some good practice with both these secondary actions.

Your goal in this introductory week is to pay attention to how your hair reacts so that you can see for yourself how it dries on its own (i.e. air-dries) from damp to fully dried and how your locks look naturally, all while familiarising yourself with the Damp vs. Dry effect and, overall, getting a good feel as to how your hair behaves without any added products or manipulation. Your mane will not look its best during this week, but take this period as a week-long lesson on your own hair. Once the week is over, shampoo your hair and perform the next step and set of actions.

## Step 4: Find out your optimal shampooing frequency and learn to style your hair

Knowing your optimal shampooing frequency is paramount. Before doing anything, have a good look at Appendix XXVI so as to get an idea of the grooming needs of your hair type.

Concentrate on finding out your optimal shampooing frequency and take your time. Use the generic guidelines as explained in Chapter 3 "Hair-Grooming Aspect: Your Daily Interacting With Your Mane" (and as also seen in Appendix XXI) during the period that you will use to find out your optimal shampooing frequency: use a normal conditioner only on your shampooing days, do the Sebum Coating method and use a leave-in conditioner on your non-shampooing days, and apply your chosen hairstyling agent every day whether it is a shampooing or non-shampooing day. Stay with only 1 hairstyling agent until you have found out your shampooing frequency.

Start practising the styling of your mane concomitantly as you find out your shampooing frequency. Familiarise yourself with your chosen hairstyling agent, get used to styling with your fingers or conventional/wide-tooth comb and grease the groove of drying your locks, whether it is with a towel or via the Shakeout method. Avoid using hair dryers for now.

Finding out your optimal shampooing frequency may take you up to 16 weeks (or even more) as you will be assessing every 2 weeks the state of your mane. Take your time, don't rush it; you will be seeing vast cosmetic improvements in your mane as you get closer to your optimal shampooing frequency.

## Step 5: Know your conditioners like you mean it

After having experienced the importance of your optimal shampooing frequency as you took the time and effort to find this particular frequency, you can now experiment with your normal conditioner frequency as well as with the frequency of use of your leave-in conditioner. Just like with shampooing frequency, give yourself some weeks to ramp up and find out your optimal frequency for both normal and leave-in conditioners although you can start using the leave-in conditioner every day without slowly ramping up the frequency if you so wish; leave-in conditioners offer great benefit when used daily as a hairstyling agent anyway.

For your normal conditioner, a good starting point is to use it on 50% of your non-shampooing days. For example, if you are doing 1 on/6 off for your shampooing frequency, then start by using the normal conditioner on 3 of those 6 "off" days (i.e. 50%); do remember though that you will also be using a normal conditioner on your shampooing day by default. This conditioner-increasing action works best for the coiled and kinky hair types.

Use the same 5 indicators used to assess your optimal shampooing frequency to now gauge and fine-tune your response to an increased conditioning frequency (normal or leave-in). Likewise, use the same trend of reviewing your hair every 2 weeks as you advance towards your optimal normal conditioning frequency, only that you will now be inserting the secondary action of "using a normal conditioner" on an extra non-shampooing day of your hair-grooming schedule. If your hair is looking too greasy, has tiny white particles breaking off or is still looking dry, then adjust the frequency of use of your normal or leave-in conditioner while leaving the shampooing frequency unaltered.

As a general rule, you will find that using a normal conditioner on your shampooing days and doing the Sebum Coating method plus using a leave-in conditioner on your non-shampooing days will, many times, suffice in terms of optimal conditioning for your mane. Thus, start with such conditioning frequencies until you secure your optimal shampooing frequency, and then, if you want to play around with a higher normal conditioner frequency, use the "50% of off days" rule; if you want to play around with a higher leave-in conditioner frequency, introduce the leave-in on 50% of those days in which it isn't used or alternatively ramp up the frequency as you desire.

## Step 6: Master the 9-Minute Perfect Mane routine

Only when you are acquainted with the 3 hair-grooming stages and their main and secondary actions, will it be time to become efficient at synchronising the stages to define your daily routine (i.e. the 9-Minute Perfect Mane routine). Basically, your goal is to master your hair-grooming routine, aiming to get to those 9 golden minutes of your daily hair-grooming time. Don't rush the process of becoming efficient with your hair-grooming routine; in the beginning, you will quite possibly take +20 minutes to finish your day's worth of hair grooming; don't worry about this. Merely worry about being determined to cut down the time that it takes you to finish your daily hair grooming, getting there slowly but surely, a few seconds less per day that passes.

The goal is to get your hair-grooming routine down to 9 minutes, not because this is the mark that defines the best-looking hair possible or because that will give you extra follicular-wizardry skills. Not at all. Getting your routine down to 9 minutes will mean that you have learnt to maximise the time-managing component of your hair grooming and can then fully reap the convenience factor of an optimal hair-management equation. For example, the 11 minutes that separate a 9-minute hair-grooming routine from a 20-minute hair-grooming routine can become crucial when you have to wake up early to go to work and you try to avoid getting stuck in rush hour traffic. And let's not forget that those 9 minutes that make up your hair-grooming routine imply not only convenience but also great-looking Is, Ss, Es or Zs.

The template for the 9-Minute Perfect Mane routine as laid out in Chapter 3 "Hair-Grooming Aspect: Your Daily Interacting With Your Mane" is the one for a typical shampooing day, which is the day that determines how the rest of your weekly schedule flows. Thus, your 9-Minute Perfect Mane routine changes secondary actions on non-shampooing days, yet the flow of stages and emphasis on the 3 main actions is at all times preserved. Always remember: you must clean, condition and style your hair regardless of the day it is.

## Step 7: Get your proactive and reactive measures sorted

The cool thing about your hair care is that you can start applying all your measures right from the very beginning of your journey; you can work on some, and you can leave others for later. However, once you have your hair-grooming routine mastered, it is time to fully address and maximise your hair-care measures and strategy.

The 2 issues of dry hair and tangled hair will already be addressed (and just about be optimised) by your hair grooming, so any added hair-care measures for these 2 issues at this point will be the icing on the cake and will integrate together with the rest of the hair-care measures that you were carrying out by default via your optimal hair grooming. Because you will have already got into the habit of optimising your mane by having addressed its grooming first, any hair-care measures that you now start implementing will too become second nature, which will possibly be in contrast to how much you dreaded these measures when you first read about them in Chapter 4 "Hair-Care Aspect: The Big 3 Issues To Battle To Sport Great-Looking Hair". For example, tying your long-length hair at this point will make much more sense and be more welcomed than when you first read about this measure.

As for hair loss, you will be noticing increased shedding due to the enhanced slip from the conditioners and your natural sebum; really, the only thing you should be doing is investing in a vacuum cleaner to remove the shed hairs from the floor.

It is also a good time to be aware of your hairline and look into your family history for any signs of male patter baldness (MPB). Part of optimising your hair-management equation is appreciating your hair and being aware of a hair-loss condition that goes with being a male, as is MPB. In Chapter 2, you will have already defined your Norwood stage, but it is now that you must really start acting if MPB seems to be taking a toll on your great-looking mane.

The advice on my nutritional approach for your hair can be applied whenever, just make sure that you stick to it long term to truly benefit from ingesting the optimal nutrients for better hair and overall health. Since this nutritional approach will affect not only the looks of your hair but also your health (for the better), you must consult your doctor prior to making any changes in your diet and/or nutritional supplementation, and it would be wise to also have a general health checkup to know your current health state and be able to compare it with any future checkups. Ask your doctor; he/she will be able to tell you what you need to do and get checked. Just like your barber or hairdresser, your doctor is another ally in your quest to own the best hair you can possibly have.

Your hair-care measures and your nutritional approach compose your hair-care strategy, or, in other words, by addressing these 2 essential elements of your hair-care aspect, you will have created the approach to looking after your hair over the long term. Your hair-care strategy is dynamic and should be reviewed from time to time; your hair-care measures will require some minor tweaks as your hair length changes over time.

It is once your hair grooming is in order and is being executed optimally that your hair care must then be fully addressed and maximised. Ultimately, these 2 aspects (hair grooming and hair care) of your hair-management equation are what will give you the great-looking hair.

## Step 8: Enhance that mane

Once you reach this step and have performed all the previous steps and necessary actions, you will have achieved the goal of great-looking hair. Anything that you do by now will consist of finishing touches because the optimal grounds for your hair-management equation will already be established.

All you have left is to give that great-looking mane a customised form and look. Trying and testing different hairstyles, choosing the right barber to get suitable haircuts, deciding whether to purchase hair accessories, merely going solo with the Shake & Go in terms of hairstyles, trying new hairstyling agents; they are all options that should be considered at this point of your journey and that are covered in Chapter 6 "Giving Your Mane Its Shape: Hairstyles, Hair Accessories, Straightening Your Locks, Growing That Mane And Getting A Haircut".

Be creative, test and experiment; hair as it is has an important experimental component that is quite awesome because each head of Is, Ss, Es and Zs is different: you will have a hair type, 2 hair lengths, a Curl Factor, a higher or lower shampooing frequency, be at whichever Norwood stage, secrete a lot or not much sebum, and, of course, there is a one and only you. The stuff that flourishes atop your head is just another piece of the puzzle that makes you, and you can most definitely use and customise this piece to your advantage; never forget that, my friend.

## **Reaching the mane-awesomeness destination**

You will have achieved your great-looking head of Is, Ss, Es or Zs when you are satisfied with your hair and with how it suits you in the grand scheme of things. The flow that I recommend for starting and developing your journey is pretty much as described in the previous section's 8 steps, but it will be you who will decide, there and then, when he is finally happy with how his hair looks. Each male differs in how he wants his hair to look, so, now that you have been shown the way, all you have left to do is to customise your hair exactly as to how you've always wanted it to look; this is, in fact, the beauty of it all, for your hair will not only look its best but will also look how you want it to peculiarly look.

Because achieving the goal of great-looking hair requires some experimenting from your part, I cannot give you a definite timespan for your journey. Approximately, you will take between 5 weeks to 17 weeks to have optimised your hair-management and be happy with your hair. The longest-taking step during your journey is the finding out of your shampooing frequency, which can take you quite a few weeks as you change the frequency every 2 weeks until you find out your optimal shampooing frequency (hence the quoted conservative figure of 17 weeks). However, and this is a big "however", you will be noticing positive results from day 1 of your journey, and the generic hair-grooming routine to be used during the finding out of your optimal shampooing frequency is made so as to have you seeing results every week during the time that it takes you to find out this crucial hair-grooming element.

With all the practice that you will get during your journey, the daily management of your hair will soon become second nature, and, when it is the time to change anything (e.g. hairstyle or shampooing frequency), you will be able to do so with no inconvenience on your part and still sporting that great mane. It is all your acquired knowledge and hands-on experience during this journey that will be determinant in having great-looking hair lifelong and without dramas. Look at it over the long term, and understand that the uniqueness of your own hair implies a certain amount of experience (i.e. your journey) prior to fully knowing and mastering those locks.

## Conclusion

The optimising of your hair-management equation is all about seeing the process as a journey in which you will be carrying out a series of actions based on steps. You must first know your hair profiling, then go on to master your hair grooming and finish by sealing the long-term life of your mane via your hair care.

The point of achieving great-looking hair is to be happy with the stuff atop your head. We all have our own definition of what "great-looking hair" is and, because this is all about customising your hair to your core self, what truly matters is that you get your hair to fit your particular understanding of aesthetic hair and you thus get to be happy with your head of Is, Ss, Es or Zs. Nothing more.

From this chapter, you should take home the message of being patient and methodical about your journey. You will start seeing improvements in your hair the moment you start your journey, yet your hair needs an experimental part that comes with the experience of managing your own hair. Worry not, you will soon have that desired great-looking mane and will be, once and for all, happy and at peace with your hair!

## Anthony's barbershop case study

Samuel was a college student with coiled hair whom Anthony had advised in person about optimising his (Samuel's) hair-management equation. The problem with Samuel was that he was all over the place; a talented artist who had received a scholarship to enrol in an art degree at college, Samuel had confessed to Anthony that he had issues with ADHD (a type of attention-deficit disorder) and that he lacked focus whenever a methodical approach was needed.

Samuel had come many times to Anthony's barbershop to get a haircut and both of them would talk about Samuel's hair-management equation all the time. However, Anthony could sense that Samuel was not getting very far with his hair management, so Anthony called me up and asked me to give him (Anthony) some pointers to pass on to Samuel so as to have Samuel finally putting order to his hair-management efforts.

I sent Anthony a list of the elements that make up each of the hair-management aspects and listed the elements in a chronological order, outlining which ones to do first. I told Anthony to give Samuel some time but that Samuel should also be reporting back to him on how he was doing. After 6 weeks, Anthony told me that Samuel had come back for a haircut and his hair had improved remarkably. Samuel had found out his shampooing frequency to be 1 on/1 off and he had stuck to the generic guideline of a normal conditioner after the shampoo on shampooing days and the Sebum Coating method and a leave-in conditioner on non-shampooing days. He had already customised his hair-grooming routine and schedule, and he was already putting to use everything concerning the hair-care aspect of his hair-management equation.

Samuel had gone back to Anthony's barbershop so as to get a new haircut for a totally-new hairstyle he had in mind for his coils. Samuel was now on the last step of his journey of putting the final touches to his mane by means of a new haircut and hairstyle. Samuel dominated already his hair profiling, hair grooming and hair care and looked like a new man (I actually met him during one of his barbershop visits). Anthony not only had a customer for life but also a friend, for Samuel was very thankful to Anthony for having changed his (Samuel's) confidence in himself via the optimal addressing of his hair-management equation.

# 8) Hair Myths: Let's Get Our Facts Straight

There are many myths and wrong beliefs surrounding hair; this being primarily engined by a lack of hair knowledge on our side (men) and by the hair-care industry having a vested interested in maintaining hair folklore alive.

Part of achieving the knowledge needed to achieve a great-looking mane is being aware of the myths that accompany hair and knowing fact from fiction. Unfortunately, many hair myths continue to be propagated in this day and age despite the advent of the internet, and there is a lot of misinformation going around with hair, especially misinformation that is then used to snowball the nonsensical mythology and folklore associated with hair. Likewise, hair-related myths are sometimes spread unintentionally by average folks while, other times, myths are spread and maintained alive by those same ones who profit from the spread of misinformation.

In this chapter, I will cover those common and not-so-common myths that surround hair and that many of us have fallen prey to at one time or another. You now have the knowledge needed to achieve the best hair that you can possibly own, but it is a fact that you will encounter some hair myths along the journey, and these myths may be tempting to fall for despite your already-extensive knowledge of your hair. So, without further ado, let's kick those myths were the sun don't shine!

## Myth 1 – Trimming hair makes it grow faster or healthier

I have heard this one even from hairdressers themselves, but it makes sense that this myth continues to be propagated as the more visits you make to the hairdresser, well, the more cash he makes. If your hairdresser tries to convince you to believe this myth, run for the hills.

The truth is that there is no way for a hair follicle to tell when the shaft has been trimmed. There is some evidence pointing to hair growing a little bit faster in summer, which is coincidentally when you are likely to get your hair trimmed more often as you will be outdoors and wanting to look good. Correlation does not imply causation, however, so cut your hair whenever you think it is optimal to do so and without factoring in this myth.

177

## Myth 2 – Shaving hair makes it grow thicker

Just like with the previous myth, the hair shaft doesn't have any nerve endings to sense when it has been shaved. Your hair follicles keep producing the same amount of hair at the same rate and with the same structure whether you shave the hair or not.

Hair that has been shaved will feel thicker when it is at a very short length (i.e. near-shaved) because the shorter a hair strand is, the less pliable it will be. Furthermore, when hair is shaved, the newly-created tip of the hair shaft is formed at an angle, which further exacerbates the perceived thickening-effect and, in effect, makes each hair strand a follicular blade knife.

Take two straws. Cut one of them so that it is only 1 inch in length while the other one remains at whatever length it is (e.g. 5 inches). Now, hold the uncut straw with one hand and use the palm of your other hand to smoothly apply pressure along the length of the straw; it will bend. Now, try to do the same on the 1-inch straw; it won't bend and will feel as though it is harder. Now, image dozens of 1-inch straws placed vertically and next to each other on a board measuring 4 inches by 4 inches. That's exactly what happens with hair as it grows after being shaved: it will go from less pliable to more pliable as the hair strands increase in length. Nothing else.

## Myth 3 – Hair grows from the tip

I have been surprised at the amount of people that I've found who think that this is true. The inclusion of this myth in this chapter is, more than anything else, to illustrate how profoundly unaware average Joes are about their hair. In the case of this myth, this is not entirely our fault as we are constantly bombarded on TV with hair products that focus solely on the ends of the hair strands, thus the association with something going on in this segment of our hair.

Good thing is that you already know that your hair grows from the follicle and that you are continuously producing new hair material, which actually provides a cushion for your hair-caring efforts because, if you end up damaging your hair, you know that new hair segments will sprout regardless. However, don't take this as green light to go and look after your hair carelessly because hair grows 0.5 inches of length per month, and any damage to the segment of the hair strands closest to the scalp can take many months to be outgrown.

## Myth 4 – Plucking 1 grey hair will have 2 growing back

Not at all. If you are lucky, the same grey hair will grow back again as if nothing happened, and, if you are unlucky, you will have damaged the hair follicle from pulling the hair strand out of the follicle socket, which will lead to defective hair growth or even no more hair growing out (grey or not grey).

My advice is to simply cut the specific grey hair strand very short with a pair of scissors if you only have a few grey hairs. If you are greying around most of your head though, then I suggest that you get on with the program: grey hair can look great and can indeed enhance your looks. On the other hand, you can dye your hair to conceal the greying but try to go with discreet and elegant tones that match your natural hair colour; don't make it too in your face.

## Myth 5 – There is good hair and there is bad hair

This myth was in part launched into the mainstream by Chris Rock's movie Good Hair although the good hair/bad hair concept has been unfairly ingrained in people with coiled and kinky hair for many decades, and, in some countries, it carries racial connotations.

The good hair/bad hair concept views coiled and kinky hair in its natural state as "bad hair" while "good hair" is viewed as hair that is either straight or wavy (albeit defined waves).

Of course, this whole good hair/bad hair thing is a lot of baloney because any man, regardless of hair type, can improve his hair substantially and thus have good hair.

In fact, if I were to dig into semantics, I would put it like this:

- "Good hair" is the equivalent of having an optimised hair-management equation.

- "Bad hair" is the equivalent of a dead rat.

179

There are no hair textures, hair types, skin tones, ethnicities or races involved when it comes to bad hair. If you don't take care of your hair, it will be "bad hair". Plain and simple.

## Myth 6 – You must shampoo your hair daily for optimal hygiene

As you know by now, the whole "shampooing daily" concept took off in the '60s with the advent of the hippie movement. As it goes, back in those days shampooing daily was cunningly associated by the big hair-care companies with not being a hippy, which helped to establish the daily use of shampoo when decades earlier, shampoo was used with lower frequencies and with less-processed ingredients.

As I have covered so enthusiastically in this book, reducing shampooing frequency is the best way to start improving your hair. From skipping shampoo every other day to shampooing once a week or even once every couple of weeks, you will have to play around a little to find out your best shampooing frequency. Make sure that you fully understand how to find out your optimal shampooing frequency and that you know what to do on the days that you do not shampoo because your optimal shampooing frequency is key in achieving great-looking hair.

## Myth 7 – You can straighten your curly hair by brushing it

Not only is this myth wrong, but, if you try it, you will end up damaging your hair. I have talked to a good number of curly men who, for some reason, believed that furiously brushing their curls like mad men would straighten their waves, coils or kinks. Then, when they saw that their hair turned into a huge ball of frizz from the brushing, they would blame their lack of results on not brushing hard enough, thus starting a vicious hair-brushing cycle that ultimately damaged their hair beyond repair. Yes, this is the extent to which many curly men are brainwashed to reject their naturally-forming curls!

If you have any of the curly hair types, brushing your hair will break its curl pattern and will only lead to merely pulling your hair and even pulling hair strands out of their follicles if you brush hard enough. Avoid at all costs.

## Myth 8 – Curly hair doesn't grow as long as straight hair

This myth is partly true. Your genetic makeup is the ultimate factor that determines the final length that your hair can achieve, and people with straight hair do not have specific genes that dictate that their hair can grow longer than curly hair. However, curly hair (be it wavy, coiled or kinky) takes the longer distance by default when it grows, and one's Curl Factor will determine how long the hair can visibly grow to (i.e. the visible length it achieves).

All factors equal (including genetic makeup), curly hair will not achieve the same final visible length that straight hair will achieve because, despite the fact that both textures will have grown to the same extended length, curly hair will have curved and bent along the way. Having said that, you should not be worrying much about this peculiarity unless you are planning to grow your hair to navel length and beyond.

## Myth 9 – Curly hair can be cut just like straight hair

As outlined in Chapter 6 "Giving Your Mane Its Shape: Hairstyles, Hair Accessories, Straightening Your Locks, Growing That Mane And Getting A Haircut", you should be striving to find a barber or hairdresser who has experience cutting your hair type, especially if your hair type falls under the curly spectrum. For the most part, curly hair must be cut in a dry state and not in a wet/damp state, which is the opposite of what a typical barber would do with straight hair (wet the hair before cutting it).

Wavy, coiled and kinky hair coils back when it dries from a wet state, and each one of us will have his unique and specific Curl Factor, which makes it almost impossible to predict how the haircut will finally look when the hair dries. Most barbers and hairdressers will not think twice before wetting curly hair and proceeding to cut it, which is the same approach that they use with straight hair.

While curly hair may be slightly dampened, especially when the majority of the cutting job has been done, you should be getting your wavy, coiled or kinky hair cut by someone who has experience cutting curly hair and who doesn't view cutting curly hair the same as cutting straight hair. You have been warned; I have experienced and seen some horrible haircut cases that stemmed from having wetted the curly hair prior to cutting it. Never underestimate the ability of your curly hair to coil back into place!

## Myth 10 – Growing your hair long makes you less predisposed to balding

I have heard this one a lot. Fact is, by having longer hair, you have a bigger mass of hair on your head, which can conceal your balding; this peculiarity being where this myth comes from. If you are balding (MPB), you should treat your hair follicles with the utmost care, so growing your mane long (6+ inches) is not the best idea as long hair has a tendency to be pulled and catch on things. Last thing you need is losing more follicular soldiers in battle through unintentional pulling. Wear your balding hair at a short or medium length, elegantly and, most of all, with pride and confidence. You can still have a decent mane as you bald; it's all about how you carry it and carry yourself!

## Myth 11 – Hair gel will make you go bald

I have heard this one so often that when I was a kid I purposely avoided hair gel like the plague. Hair gel will not make you go bald since baldness in men is caused by a specific androgen hormone (dihydrotestosterone) and your scalp's sensitivity to its effects. Having said that, some hair gels are choked with so many artificial ingredients that you are best choosing hair gels with a sensible amount of ingredients, only because some shady manufacturers throw in some ingredients that may not be 100% safe in the long run.

## Myth 12 – Wearing a cap will make you go bald

Another myth that seems to be rampant among young dudes, and which is fuelled by parents unknowingly, is the one about how wearing caps will suffocate one's hair and make one go bald.

I have already written the following in the hair gel myth, but, with myth busting, there's no such thing as overemphasising: balding is caused primarily by DHT and one's unique response to the hormone's effect at the hair-follicle level. Your hair strands don't breathe, so the fact that your hair is covered by a cap doesn't mean that the hair strands, or even the hair follicles, will suffocate. Your hair follicles obtain all their essential nutrients internally, and you'd have to be wearing a tightly-sealed, air-tight, vacuum-packed cap and go malnourished for months at a time to even begin to worry about "suffocating" the skin in your scalp (ultimately leading to hair loss).

The real reason, as with most myths, is that correlation does not imply causation. Many men (especially those in their 20s) who happen to start balding prematurely tend to wear caps to hide their balding. Since male pattern baldness can progress rapidly and without one (and others) noticing its effects until the balding is in an advanced state, the wearing of a cap can disguise the true extent of the balding that is taking place. Then, it is very easy to blame it on the cap.

One thing, though: wearing a cap (or a hat) too frequently and too tight can damage the hair strands across the area of the scalp where the cap is fitted. This occurs from the mechanical friction of fitting the cap itself, which can lead to hair breaking off or, in extreme cases, manifest itself as localised and reversible bald patches. You'd have to be a massive cap enthusiast to have to worry about this though, and the best thing that you can do is to not fit yours caps or hats too tight.

## Myth 13 – Baldness is inherited from the mother's side

No. Research has shown that, while baldness can be inherited from the mother's side, baldness can also be inherited from the father's side. My advice to you is to research your family tree and see if any of the males in both sides of your family line have had male pattern baldness (go back 2 or even 3 generations).

Be aware that, if any of the recent males in your family have gone bald before the age of 35, you will have a higher risk of developing MPB. Keep an eye out and ask around.

## Myth 14 – Sun exposure speeds up hair loss

Having lived in sunny countries throughout my life, I have come across this myth quite a lot. Of course, sun exposure does not accelerate hair loss, and there are, in fact, 2 reasons for this myth.

The first reason explaining this myth is that, in someone with dark hair and with a fair-skinned balding scalp, tanning will conceal the remaining hair strands on the scalp because the skin will have darkened from the sun exposure. Dark hair is more visible on fair skin than on dark skin, and strong sun exposure, even at high latitudes, will quickly tan a balding scalp, thus giving the impression that there is less hair than otherwise.

The second reason explaining this myth is that sun exposure is associated with deterioration of the skin. This is partly true in that excessive sun exposure (think, going on holiday to the beach and getting sunburnt) will damage the skin and create a wrinkly, leathery appearance if excessive sun exposure occurs over the span of many years. However, there's no direct link between sun exposure and the speeding up of hair loss or balding; people have automatically assumed that because sun exposure is bad for the skin, it must also be bad for hair loss (i.e. augment it). Mind you and in any case, it is excessive and ridiculous sun exposure that damages the skin; the right amount of sun exposure is actually healthy and stimulates the skin!

## Myth 15 – You can train your hair to be a certain shape or type

Your hair grows from your follicles as genetically determined, hence you have your given hair type. While hair texture/type can change at critical stages of one's life (e.g. puberty), your hair will not otherwise change how it grows just because you think you are training it. Last time I checked, for something to be trained, it needs to be able to assimilate information, process it and learn from it. You can train your dog to fetch your slippers, but you certainly cannot train your hair to grow wavy instead of kinky. Of course, you can make the most of your hair and turn it into an awesome head of Is, Ss, Es or Zs, but that implies solely making your hair looks the best it can within your identified hair type.

Critical stages of one's life in which hair can change its hair type or texture include puberty, entering seniorhood, extreme distress (e.g. loss of a loved one), going through cancer treatment and taking some very-specific medications that are used for serious illnesses.

## Myth 16 – Men who care after their hair are girly or effeminate

I have heard this one especially from those men sporting dead rats for hair. These same men believe that taking care of your hair means spending half of your morning in the bathroom putting all kinds of potions on your hair while baking a cake in the oven as you make time to watch repeat episodes of <u>Sex in the City</u>. Yeah, right.

Sure, in the beginning, you will take a bit of time (nothing major though) and will require some weeks to have everything on auto-pilot, but that's because you're starting from zero and from years of either neglecting your hair or doing everything wrong! As it goes, I have made it my personal goal in this book to never put you in a position where you have to sacrifice your testosterone levels or manhood in the name of great-looking hair.

Oh, and women love men with great-looking hair and despise dead rats. Next time you hear a dead-rat owner say nonsense like this, smile at him as you grab your beautiful lady by the derriere and kiss her in the cheek. Hey, perhaps he'll get inspired!

## Myth 17 – For males, hair cannot be managed properly no matter what and is an overall annoyance to have

Yes, I have left this one till the end. Booting this myth is pretty much the essence of this book. I remember going to hairdressers and being told to either spend my money on a silly hairstyle that would last 1 day or to go for a buzz cut or a short neat trim; same goes for barbers in barbershops. It wasn't until I decided to experiment plentifully with my hair and the hair of others that I found out that hair can look great and be conveniently managed so long as one abides by a method and a system and is capable of seeing the overall picture as well as see the need to implement every hair-management action holistically.

As a male, hair can indeed be an annoyance and be difficult to live with; the same way that driving a car can also be annoying and difficult if you have to drive a tin-looking car that is falling apart and you don't know how to drive it. Yet, upgrade to a Lamborghini Gallardo Superleggera (gee, I love this car) and learn how to drive it, and the driving experience then becomes pleasurable and is something that you can incorporate nicely into your lifestyle so as to have a more convenient and enjoyable life. The same concept applies to a male's hair, and the awesome thing is that you now know how to make the existence of your mane a pleasurable one and are consequently able to reap its cosmetic and lifestyle benefits.

## Conclusion

There's a lot of misinformation surrounding hair and its management. There are many small-time myths and pretty much anyone can come up with a myth from having first gathered sufficient amounts of misinformation. It only takes your neighbour's wife to say that her cousin heard his son's teacher say that black-haired children are noisier in class than blonde-haired children to then snowball the initial nonsense and inflate the amount of "heard-it-through-the-grapevine" garbage that can quickly spread as people continue to gossip; the internet is a double-edged sword when it comes to this, and many times it (the internet) actually does more bad than good.

As you achieve and continue with your great-looking head of Is, Ss, Es or Zs, you will encounter myths that will be about hair loss, hair growth, hair management or that will associate weird traits to particular hair types. My advice is to always go back to this book, and, if I haven't covered this myth per se or haven't addressed in the book the topic that the myth is about, chances are that you're dealing with just another silly piece of folklore.

My goal with this book is to not only teach you all about your hair but to also have you understanding it, to have you knowing not just the whats and hows but also the whys. Thus, do use this book whenever you come across a myth but do also use common sense. If someone claims that putting banana peels on your scalp makes your hair glossier, then ask yourself, what would be the process by which banana peels, whatever may be in them, would actually make my hair strands glossier? That said, none of us are perfect, and you may still fall for a myth here and there; don't sweat it, just brush it off and continue managing your hair as established.

# Anthony's barbershop case study

Frankie was a 20-something-years-old aspiring actor (he always hid his real age like all good actors do!) who had coiled hair. He had been coming to Anthony's barbershop for years and was a regular client. Frankie preferred to keep his coils at a short length (1-2 inches) and would always look polished. Out of a sudden, Frankie stopped his regular monthly visits; Anthony had noticed this, but thought that Frankie could have very well decided to change barbers, so Anthony didn't think much of it.

A year later, Anthony randomly bumped into Frankie in the street. Frankie's hair looked different as it was long and looked unhealthy, to the point that Anthony didn't recognise Frankie at first sight. It turns out that Frankie had stopped going to Anthony's barbershop so as to grow his hair long; in that whole year, he hadn't trimmed or cut his hair. However, it turned out that Frankie was growing his hair specifically, despite the fact that he hated long hair, because he had heard from a friend, whom at the same time had read in a men's magazine, that long-haired men don't suffer from male pattern baldness (MPB); a silly blank statement that is as big of a myth as Big Foot is. MPB was very common in Frankie's family, so, as an actor, Frankie feared he'd go bald; thus his 1-year-long futile crusade against MPB in the form of growing his hair long.

Anthony calmed Frankie down and assured him that there was no need to continue growing his hair long just because he (Frankie) thought (erroneously) that longer hair would protect him from MPB. Anthony had a quick look at Frankie's scalp and told him (Frankie) that he still had the same bushy coiled mane that he used to have back when he'd hit Anthony's barbershop for a trim every month. The next day, Frankie was back in Anthony's barbershop with a smile and ready for a much-needed haircut that was long awaited!

# 9) Questions & Answers: The Miscellaneous Stuff You Will Ask Yourself

If you have got to this chapter, you will have already acquired all the knowledge necessary to take your hair from a dreaded dead rat or forced buzz cut to an awesome mane. By now, you know which hair type and hair lengths you have, what a conditioner is, what hair grooming entails, how to go about your hair care, and you will already be stoked to master the 9-Minute Perfect Mane routine. You will be exuding heaps of positivity about starting your journey, and you will be on your way to joining our ranks of dudes with great heads of Is, Ss, Es and Zs. I can assure you that you are about to boost your potential as a $21^{st}$ century male once you start putting everything into practice and get ready to achieve your particular set of great-looking, convenient hair.

Of course, as the journey to mane awesomeness starts, questions will arise. Most of these questions can be solved by referring back to the previous chapters, yet there are some other minor questions that may arise as your journey continues and that require to be specifically addressed somewhere in this book. Since I have been in your very same place, I know that there will be times when questions will indeed arise. Let's tackle them.

## 1) Why should I strive for better hair?

What, you are asking this at this stage?

Ok, joking aside. You will ask yourself this question a couple of times in the beginning, and you may have already asked yourself this very same as you continued reading this book. Your answer to this question should be, "because I want to do it".

You want to strive for and achieve a great-looking mane because, as a man, you want to make the most of what you have; you now have the right knowledge and the right mentality to fix a trait of yours that has so much potential. Before, you could excuse your way out of doing something about your Is, Ss, Es or Zs, but now there's no escaping this. And there is no escaping this because, now that you have seen the light, you can set and follow the right path.

You are now able to strive towards a better head of hair with ease and do something positive about a unique trait of yours that is part of who you are as a whole. You can buzz your mane, you can grow it long, you can style it in a myriad of ways, and you can shampoo it once or twice a week; it doesn't matter. What matters is that now you know how to make the most of something that is written in your DNA and that is inherent to you. All this without the inconvenience and associated nonsense that you once thought was synonym of sporting great-looking hair as a male.

## 2) How long will it take me to be ultimately happy with my hair?

Subjectively, as soon as you finish reading this book. Objectively, it can take you up to 4 months (roughly).

Depending on how much of a dead rat or a buzz cut you have, doing everything as outlined in this book will have you noticing visible and tangible awesome mane results in as little as a week, but I rather give you a conservative time period of up to 17 weeks since I don't know the specific circumstances surrounding your mane, nor can I know your mindset and readiness. From my experience with others though, up to 17 weeks is all it takes unless the finding of your optimal shampooing frequency is delayed severely.

Because having great-looking hair requires you to master the advice in this book so as to have your hair doing as you want it to and not vice versa, the optimising of your hair-management equation will require an initial period of learning and adapting that will consist of a few weeks. However, do not rush your adaptation, and see this for the long term; it took me years to learn all of this on my own and fully customise my own head of Es, so I have weeded out all the unnecessary stuff that I went through, and a couple of weeks will pass by fast anyway. What matters is that, as soon as you have finished reading this book, you will be en route to having the great hair that you used to dream about but never thought was possible!

### 3) What if I cannot get down to 9 minutes with my hair-grooming routine?

Nothing. Absolutely nothing will happen.

The 9 minutes of the ideal hair-grooming routine is a mark of time maximisation and efficiency; 9 minutes as a timespan for one's hair grooming is perfectly doable by any able-bodied male, and it's in your interest to work towards gradually lowering your hair-grooming time until you are under 9 minutes.

If you find that you cannot get down to 9 minutes for whatever reason, you will still be the owner of a great head of hair, provided that you do the rest of your hair management as outlined in this book. You will have certainly excelled at synchronising your hair-grooming routine if you can get it all done under 9 minutes, but there's more to great-looking hair than taking this or that long to groom your hair every day. Moreover, your hair grooming may take longer than 9 minutes on some days despite the fact that you are good at it and can normally get it all done in less than 9 minutes. We all, from time to time, like to enjoy showering for more than 9 minutes with warm water and singing rock hits from the '80s!

In conclusion, just keep in mind that the 9 minutes for your hair-grooming time is a mere objective cue that will tell you that you have become sufficiently efficient in your hair grooming and that you can then fully milk the whole convenience factor your hair-management equation. That's all.

### 4) What if I don't shower in the morning, how should I do my hair-grooming routine?

If you don't shower in the morning, then you can do the day's worth of your hair-grooming routine later in the day when you shower (e.g. after the gym); if you are showering before going to bed, then there is no point in styling your hair although there is certainly a point in cleaning and conditioning your hair. Since it is in the morning when you will typically style your hair, what you'll then do is wet your hair in the morning to style it and do your cleaning and conditioning later in the day when you have more time (e.g. during the pre-bed shower).

The hair-grooming process should ideally be implemented sequentially and without a break; that is, the stages should follow each other smoothly as per the 9-Minute Perfect Mane routine. However, if you find yourself not being able to get the 3 stages implemented in one go, then it is fine to break them up so that you carry out each stage at different times of the day. Likewise, the hair-grooming process is best done in the shower as it is more convenient although you can implement it elsewhere too (e.g. using water from the sink basin).

## 5) What if I miss a day of my hair-grooming routine?

Ideally, you should be striving to complete the hair-grooming process every day. However, we cannot ensure that we clean, condition and style our manes every single day for the rest of our lives. A day here and there without grooming your hair won't have any effects, but, if you start skipping days, you will certainly start to see a decrease in the good looks of your hair. Same goes for your hair-care strategy: regularly skipping its daily doing will negatively affect the health of your hair.

The cool thing about our hair-grooming routine is that, if you are going to be showering within the day, you can implement the grooming of your hair easily and without any inconvenience. Moreover, your hair grooming is easy to pair up with the rest of your body grooming and you'll be able to do it all in minutes. Your hair grooming will soon become second nature, and you will get to associate a quick shower with getting your mane groomed optimally.

## 6) Which should I do first, my hair grooming or my body grooming?

It is up to you. However, the 9-Minute Perfect Mane routine, as outlined for your shampooing day, takes into account that you do your body grooming in the 2 minutes that are used to leave the conditioner on your hair, and 2 minutes is more than enough to get your body groomed (i.e. cleaned).

Preferably, do your body grooming before your hair grooming on your non-shampooing days and also on your shampooing days if your body grooming happens to take more than 2 minutes. This body-grooming preference is only so as to not interrupt the flow between the conditioning and styling stages of your hair-grooming routine.

Lastly, any facial shaving should be done after your styling stage, not before.

## 7) What ingredients should I look for in a shampoo and the 2 conditioners?

Your shampoo should have at least 1 sulfate-type ingredient. These are some common names that sulfate-type ingredients can go by:

- Sodium laureth sulfate

- Sodium lauryl sulfate

- Sodium lauryl ether sulfate

- Sodium dodecyl sulfate

- Sodium monolauryl sulfate

There are also shampoos that are sulfate free, but my advice is to first start with a sulfate-based shampoo, finding out your optimal shampooing frequency and building your hair-grooming routine with such a shampoo. Then, once you are finally happy with your newly-achieved mane, you can try a sulfate-free shampoo and see how it goes. Sulfate-free shampoos are weaker than sulfate-based shampoos in their hair-cleaning action, hence it is better that you start your follicular journey using the latter as sulfate-based shampoos tend to be more common and are more convenient to use when initially finding out your optimal shampooing frequency.

For your clarifying shampoo, just go by the product name including the word "clarifying" in the label; most of these shampoos contain a sulfate-type ingredient plus other specific hair-cleaning ingredients.

With regards to your normal and leave-in conditioners, you should be identifying in their ingredient list at least 1 of the following commonly-added ingredients:

- Glycerol

- Propylene glycol

- Glyceryl stearate

- Cetearyl alcohol

- Cetyl alcohol

- Stearyl alcohol

- Glycerine

There are many functional ingredients that both normal and leave-in conditioners can have, but the ingredients listed above are the common ones used to make hair-conditioning products. Thus, when purchasing your 2 types of conditioners, aim to buy those that have at least 1 of the ingredients from the list above.

## 8) How are ingredients listed in hair products? Do they follow any pattern?

The ingredient list of every hair product comes in a descending order of ingredient predominance, thus each ingredient present in the product appears in the ingredient list as determined by its relative weight in the formula of the product: the ingredient that is most present in the product (by weight) will therefore be listed first (i.e. at the top of the list) whereas the least-present ingredient in the product will be listed last (i.e. at the bottom of the list).

Be aware that, instead of being listed vertically (i.e. from top to bottom), the ingredients present in a hair product may be listed horizontally from left to right in the ingredient list. Ergo, since the ingredient lists of hair products are always in descending order of predominance, in the case of horizontally-listed ingredients, the most-present ingredient in the product will begin as the first ingredient on the left of the ingredient list and, from there onwards, the descending order of the products will be manifested as the listing of the remaining ingredients towards the right. In the case that there are several lines conforming the ingredient list, it will be the ingredient listed on the left of the first line that starts off the descending order. The ingredient following in descending order from the last product listed in the first line (i.e. appearing furthest to the right) will thus begin as the ingredient furthest to the left in the second line.

Ideally you want to have the specific ingredients that provide the claimed benefit of the hair product listed as high (or as further to the left) as possible, for this will mean that the product is rich in the ingredients that it claims to benefit from and that are claimed to give the product its oomph. The exception to this occurs when the desired ingredients are very potent (i.e. minute amounts are needed to yield the desired benefit), which will mean that, despite being present in the product in the right amounts, the ingredients will still appear listed at the end. Some hair-product ingredients do function at minimal quantities, and a big increase in their normal presence in a product can still comprise a tiny amount of presence in the overall product.

With regards to shampoos and conditioners, the ingredients listed in Question 7 should appear at the beginning of the ingredient list. Most commonly, water (aka "aqua" when listed as an ingredient) appears as the first ingredient in shampoos and conditioners, but water should then be followed in the ingredient list by a (or several) sulfate-type ingredient in the case of shampoos or by one (or several) of the hair-conditioning ingredients in Question 7 for conditioners (both normal and leave-in conditioners).

With regards to other hair products aside from shampoos and conditioners, the ingredients are always listed as aforementioned: by descending order of predominance. However, the active ingredients (i.e. the ingredients that carry out the claimed benefit of the product) may appear towards the end of the list and not at the beginning due to being very potent in relation to their weight.

## 9) Why is my hair type coiled or kinky when it is short, yet looks wavy when it is long?

Your hair follicles keep producing the same hair type regardless of your hair length, and there are no nerve endings in the shaft to allow the follicle to sense when the hair is long enough to change its texture.

This noticeable curl-smoothing effect that you and the rest of curly dudes experience when their hair is long is due to the weighting down of the hair once the curls reach a long-enough length, with this effect being most noticeable on long coiled hair. Because of the inherent weight of long hair, the hair closest to the scalp will be pulled down continuously, leaving the curls in this segment of the strands in a permanent semi-extended state. Thus, the curls formed in the segment of the hair strands closest to the scalp will look smoother and looser in curl shape than the curls formed closer to the tip. On the other hand, the ends (i.e. tips) of curly hair don't have any extra length to weight them down, so it is this segment of the hair locks that resembles what one's true hair shape is.

Note that this effect is most relevant when your hair starts to hang down naturally without hairstyling agents applied, which tends to be at the visible lengths of 4 inches for straight hair, 4 to 6 inches for wavy hair, and 8+ inches for coiled and kinky hair.

## 10) Why does my wavy, coiled or kinky hair look awkward when I try to grow it long?

The 3 curly hair types are known for growing in an awkward manner, especially when the hair is grown carelessly (i.e. the opposite of how you'll be doing as per this book). If you happen to have curly hair, you quite likely have tried in the past to grow your curls to a long length but found that your hair would look worse the longer it grew. This awkward phase tends to last until the curls get to hang down naturally, thus a curly male growing his mane long can stay with awkward-looking hair for 1-3 years at a time, and most males can't make it that long and prefer to chop their hair before having to endure the drama of growing beastly hair.

If you want to grow your curls long, the best thing that you can do is to start from a hair length that is fairly even all around your head. The length difference between the longest and the shortest hair segments on your scalp should be a maximum of 2 inches. For example, if your hair has been trimmed with the sides and back of your head shorter than the top and you want to grow your hair long (over 6 inches), then you'd want the hair on the top of your head to not be longer than 2 inches from the hair on the sides and back of your head.

The awkwardness of curly hair when growing it long is primarily due to this texture's inherent puffing-out nature, and having uneven hair lengths will magnify the puffing out and thus create said awkwardness. Growing your hair via your optimised hair-management equation will make growing your curls long a piece of cake, but it won't fully protect you from having to endure some hair awkwardness before your curls get to fully hang down.

## 11) I want to grow my hair long, how will I be seen by society (especially at work)?

Society as a whole has a negative view on men with long hair. This view stems from the rebellious character that long hair has been traditionally associated with. From hippies to rock stars, long hair exudes rebellion, alternative thinking, nonconformism and possibly sex addiction! Of course, in today's corporate-driven society, this rebellious image is frowned upon because your boss doesn't want the girls in the office lusting and daydreaming about your long locks; talk about diminished productivity!

Having spoken with several human resources directors over the years and spending much of my career in a corporate environment, I can vouch for the negative view on men with long hair. Mind you, I have managed to pull long hair in my career because I have made sure to have a polished and professional image so as to neutralise the prejudiced perspective on long hair; a feat that is easier said than done. Moreover, curly hair has it worst when it comes to pulling it off at work as curly hair already has a rebellious nature associated to it due to its inherent "beast that can't be tamed" factor, so having long hair as a curly dude is a very delicate matter.

If your job is in a corporate or conservative environment and you want to grow your hair long, all I can tell you is to really work on your image and totally master the 9-Minute Perfect Mane routine. This means to never look scruffy, dirty or unkempt because, if you do, your long hair will be the icing on the cake for your work colleagues to start regarding you as an unprofessional individual. Quite a few men approach the growing of their manes with a carefree attitude that is not optimal for a modern male like you and I. Long hair will add a lot to your looks and will benefit you greatly only if you have a polished image, so think of long hair as a magnifying glass: it can make you look better or worse depending on how well groomed and cared your mane is.

## 12) I am trying to do the Sebum Coating method, but I am uncertain about grabbing locks of hair, can you explain further what I should be doing?

Unless you have a very low hair density, you will have discernible locks: a number (ranging from a dozen to a few dozens) of hair strands will be growing in the same direction, effectively forming locks, and thus being easy to spot on the scalp. If you run your hands through your hair, you will be able to tell apart these locks as the hair strands group together and form visible "chunks" of hair. Basically, you could say that your mane is made up of many hair locks growing from your scalp, for each hair lock is made up of individual hair strands grouped together.

Sometimes, the locks are not so easy to tell, this being most common in straight hair and very tight kinky hair. If you find that you cannot tell your locks apart, worry not, for having "visible" locks is more of an interesting occurrence than anything else; it doesn't mean that your hair needs to be managed any differently. In the case that your hair strands don't seem to clump into locks, simply grab as much hair as you can in 1-inch-wide sets and run your fingers through the sets as described for the Sebum Coating method. Effectively, someone who has visible locks will be grabbing 3-10 locks at a time in each 1-inch-wide set, yet you'll be grabbing just as much hair in each set, only that you won't be grabbing what would otherwise be locks (since your hair strands don't grow grouped as locks). In any case, this is a mere semantic issue; whether your hair strands group into visible locks or not, simply grab as much hair as you can in 1-inch-wide sets to implement the Sebum Coating method.

## 13) Is working on my hair going to negatively affect my masculinity?

No, no and no! While I understand your concern about having your masculinity sacrificed in the name of great-looking hair, the reality is that the vast majority of dudes that we see around with buzz cuts haven't done anything about their manes because they all lack inspiration and knowledge.

These same aforementioned men with their insignia buzz cuts have experienced the dead-rat effect previously; they have had bad experiences with their hair and, overall, don't know how to properly go about their Is, Ss, Es and Zs, so they automatically have a negative feeling towards their hair and prefer to forget about it by hitting the barber for a close crop every 2 weeks. This is quite a natural response: if you regard something as bad or negative, you are not going to do something about it unless you are shown the proper and optimal way to do it or fix it.

With this book, you get all your hair knowledge and you get to insert this knowledge into your daily life in a convenient manner. I am the first one who avoids colourful hair salons with teacups everywhere, Mickey-Mouse stuff and wasting my time and hard-earned money on hair minutiae: I go about my life with my mane addressed optimally and conveniently, no muss no fuss. Thus, I now pass on to you all my knowledge so that you too can do the same and can start regarding the stuff atop your head as an enhancement to your life. For all intents and purposes, your masculinity will actually be enhanced with your optimised hair, not impaired.

## 14) Can you go into more detail with guard lengths?

Guard lengths are the lengths of hair to which hair is cropped at with a hair clipper. A hair clipper is a tool that you will have seen your barber use to crop your hair very short and for which there are adjustable guards that allow the choosing of a specific length to crop the hair at. You can buy a hair clipper for yourself to use since this device is helpful in maintaining certain hairstyles that require frequent trims.

There are several manufacturers of hair clippers in the market, and some may use slightly different numbers for their guard lengths, but, on average, they stick to the following guard lengths:

- **#1:** 0.125 inches (3 millimetres)

- **#2:** 0.250 inches (6 millimetres)

- **#3:** 0.375 inches (9 millimetres)

- **#4:** 0.5 inches (13 millimetres)

Guard lengths under a #1 are also available, and different manufacturers approach their numbering differently. Don't overcomplicate it though as the length differences between guard lengths under a #1 are in 0.05 inches intervals, so, if you decide to purchase a hair clipper, just choose one that goes from a #0 up to a #4 and has the option of cropping shorter than a #0.

## 15) Why does it look like I shed more now that I use conditioners?

On average, males shed approximately 100 hair strands per day. This is a natural and normal process of the scalp, and it is part of the life cycle of each hair strand. A hair strand goes through a growth cycle that can last up to 8 years (it is genetically determined), and, once this growth cycle is completed, the hair strand detaches itself from the follicle (i.e. sheds) and typically falls off in the same moment. However, sometimes the shed hair strands may become trapped in the curves and bends that make up the rest of one's unshed hair strands. This is very common with curly hair, and every day you walk around with shed hair trapped in your mane that will eventually fall off or be removed intentionally or unintentionally with a comb or your fingers.

Both normal and leave-in conditioners add extra slip to your hair, which is why these products are great for avoiding hair tangles. Due to the extra slip provided by conditioners, you will find that the shed hair strands, which in the past would get trapped in the rest of your growing hair strands, will now be falling off and be removed easily, both when you style your mane and when you are just going about your day. You will very likely notice more hairs than usual being removed during your grooming as soon as you start using conditioners and optimising your hair-grooming routine, and this can be mistaken for unnatural hair loss. Unless your hairline is receding or you notice a marked decrease in hair density on your scalp, you have absolutely nothing to worry about.

## 16) Why does it look like I shed more when my hair is long?

Just like mistaking shed hairs for unnatural hair loss or balding when you start using conditioners, you may also fall for misinterpreting the natural shedding process when you grow your hair to a length that you have never had it before.

The reason for thinking that you are shedding more when your hair is longer is because you have more hair, plain and simple! I remember freaking out when I first grew my mane to a very long length (15 inches) and realised that the longer my hair grew, the more I seemed to be shedding, which of course was of worry as it could mean that I was starting to bald. The thing is, despite many years have passed since I first freaked out, I still have the same bushy head of Es that I used to rock back in those days (touch wood, though!). Really, you will notice more shed hairs because there is more hair material to be physically seen.

## 17) Why all the confusion about hair density?

Many people mistake how full and bushy one's hair may look with how dense it is. Hair density actually refers to how many hair strands one has per centimetre square of skin. In the scalp, this figure varies between 150 to 250 hair strands per centimetre square, and the average male has anywhere from 90,000 to 140,000 hair strands in his scalp. One can easily have a high hair density yet not have his mane looking full and bushy, and the reverse is also true: one can have a low hair density and still appear to have a full and bushy mane.

This fullness effect is caused by one's Curl Factor, the actual thickness of each individual hair strand and how long the hair is. Thus, those with coiled and kinky hair who grow their manes to long lengths will appear to have very full and bushy manes as opposed to those with straight and wavy hair.

In conclusion, the take-home message is that dense hair is hair that has a high number of hair strands per square centimetre.

## 18) When will my hair hang down?

The hanging down of one's hair is a milestone that many guys look forward to. Your mane can be made to hang down artificially before it will hang down naturally by using a leave-in conditioner as your hairstyling foundation and then adding a styling cream on top (of the leave-in). Basically, you want to add extra weight to the hair strands to encourage the weighting down of your locks, and this is best done by using these 2 aforementioned hairstyling agents together.

However, for your hair to hang down naturally (i.e. in a dried state and with no hair products applied), these are the approximate visible hair lengths (not extended lengths!) that you will need:

- **Straight hair:** 4 inches (will start to hang down at 2 inches)

- **Wavy hair:** 6 inches (will start to hang down at 4 inches)

- **Coiled hair:** 10 inches (will start to hang down at 6-8 inches)

- **Kinky hair:** 15+ inches (will start to hang down at 10 inches)

Again, the above hair lengths are visible lengths, not extended lengths. Take into account that very-curly kinky hair may virtually never get to fully hang down, especially the hair on the top of the head. If you have kinky hair and want your mane to fully hang down, then it is best that you braid or lock your hair.

I would recommend you to not obsess about your hair hanging down. The above timespans are conservative (as with all growth estimations for hair), and, for the most part, your hair will have to be at a long (extended) length to fully hang down. Instead of obsessing about this minute aspect of your already-achieved great-looking mane, focus on finding the right hairstyle for your hair type and embracing that which comes to you naturally.

# 19) Why do my curls puff out so much?

This is not only a good question but also a very common question that I get from curly dudes. First of all, the curving and bending nature of curly hair naturally predisposes this hair texture to puff out; that's the way it is, and, the sooner you accept this, the better. Your curly hair (be it wavy, coiled or kinky) will continue to puff out until it reaches a length that it can hang down as per the previous question. Essentially, there is a period of length, which commonly falls under the medium-length category and is what I called the "awkward phase", where the hair will puff out the longer it grows until it hits the specific length in which it will hang down.

The good news is that your curly hair will puff out, correct, but it will puff out awesomely through the hair-equation system. Your curls will be tamed and the puffing out will be controlled via your optimal hair grooming and hair care that you have learnt as part of optimising your hair-management equation. Don't view puffy hair as bad; curly men have been brainwashed to buzz their curls and straighten their hair, and you and I know very well that that's not what you will be doing once you achieve your great-looking mane of Ss, Es or Zs. If your hair continues to puff out once you achieve your mane-awesomeness goal, then so be it: you are taking good care of your hair and you are managing it daily, and that's what matters.

Like I say, your optimal hair-management equation will have you controlling your puffiness, but you must bear in mind that curly hair is innately puffy albeit with different ranges according to one's particular hair strands. Thus, achieve your goal of being happy with your hair, and walk proud with those luxuriant curls, even if they puff out!

# 20) Why is my hair type different now from when I was a boy?

Many men find that their current adult hair type is different from the hair type they had as boys. This is believed to be due to the effect that the puberty-induced increase in levels of sex hormones has on the development of hair follicles although the precise mechanism of action for this is not known. After puberty, a big percentage of males move up in hair type instead of moving down (e.g. from wavy to coiled).

My beast was a beautiful, soft and bouncy mane of waves when I was child. Then, I hit puberty, and my hair turned into a bushy beast of coils and kinks; I also transformed heavily all over my body, so the transformation of my hair was one of my lesser worries (I had a beard at age 12 that all the older guys in my school were jealous of).

## 21) Can I shampoo daily?

Yes, you can, especially if you have near-shaved hair. Even if you have longer hair, you can shampoo daily, but my advice to you is to then use a sulfate-free shampoo or weaker hair-cleaning products if you want to shampoo daily. Bear in mind that you will have to adapt your hair-grooming schedule to this preference in shampooing frequency.

## 22) What if my hair gets very dirty due to a specific occasion?

If your hair gets very dirty from a specific occasion such as going camping or being in a closed room where people smoke, you can then schedule a shampooing session and treat the session as if it were a shampooing day (i.e. follow the shampooing with normal conditioner and style with your hairstyling agent). Resume your normal shampooing frequency the next day; that is, you will have restarted your weekly schedule with the previous day's shampooing.

If, on the other hand, you get your hair dirty on an occasional basis or in a frequent manner, then adapt your shampooing frequency to such. A typical scenario is playing contact sports such as wrestling: you'd certainly want to shampoo your hair after a wrestling session or any other contact-sport session. On the other hand, you don't need to shampoo if all you have done is gone to the gym and haven't rubbed your head against benches or mats. So long as your hair isn't rubbing against anything dirty, you don't have to schedule specific shampooing sessions.

If you go to the swimming pool, then I advise you to treat that day as a shampooing day; thus, deem such an activity as a hair-dirtying one since chlorine from the swimming pool is left as residue on your hair. A trick that has worked for me and for those who have tried it under my advice is to, before jumping in the swimming pool, first completely wet your hair with tap water (e.g. from the shower next to the swimming pool) and then rapidly coat your hair in conditioner (with either a normal or leave-in conditioner); you'll then be ready to hit the pool. I find a leave-in conditioner is more convenient for this trick as you can buy some leave-in conditioners in spray form or small-package form. After the swimming pool, try to do the hair-grooming process (as a shampooing day) before your hair dries completely from the pool's water. This same trick applies to seawater too (e.g. going to the beach), although you can skip the wetting of hair with tap water and the soaking with conditioner since seawater is much less harsher than swimming-pool water (simply do a shampooing session once you get home from the beach).

As an alternative method to using shampoo for the above, you may use baking soda and vinegar to clean your hair on those specific occasions that your hair has got dirty. The method itself to using baking soda and vinegar as cleaning agents is detailed in Questions 33, but, in a nutshell, you can clean your hair with baking soda and then with vinegar (instead of with shampoo) for such specific hair-dirtying days, and you don't need to follow the baking soda/vinegar with a normal conditioner (just move on to your styling stage when the vinegar is rinsed).

## 23) My hair gets too oily even with a shampooing frequency of 1 on/1 off, what should I do?

From my experience, any male who finds his hair too oily 24 hours after shampooing is either using too much hairstyling agent/s or not doing the Sebum Coating method correctly.

Use less of the hairstyling agent you may be using and try to stick to lighter agents, such as hair gel, mousse or pomade (even try water-soluble hairstyling agents, see Question 34). Likewise, aim to work your Sebum Coating method efficiently and follow the precise instructions you've learnt in this book as well as get practising. Lastly, you may use a baking soda/vinegar rinse (refer to Question 33) to clean your hair 24 hours after shampooing and then go back to shampooing the day after the baking soda/vinegar rinse so that you are effectively doing a 1 on/1 off shampooing frequency (you use the baking soda/vinegar on your "off" days).

In the rare event that your hair still becomes too oily after 24 hours, then, by all means, shampoo; even if it means having to shampoo every day.

## 24) Do I have to use nutritional supplements together with my diet?

Not at all. Nutritional supplements are only recommended so as to bulletproof your diet and have an optimal nutritional approach. Because nutrition is so important to sustain an optimal and healthy growing of hair strands, supplements allow you to provide nutrients to your hair that you aren't otherwise providing in sufficient quantities via your diet. One of the disadvantages of being a modern male is that, many times, we don't eat the healthiest and most nutrient-dense foods, thus nutritional supplements are very useful so as to make sure that we are not running low on any nutrients needed by the body and the follicles.

Overall, the most important part of your nutritional approach is your diet, not your supplementation, and you can certainly skip the use of nutritional supplements.

## 25) Isn't whey protein a steroid or dangerous?

No. Whey protein has been given a bad reputation because it is used by bodybuilders to up their daily protein intake. Bodybuilders already have a bad reputation, as it is, for taking steroids (another myth; not all take steroids), thus anything that they ingest is deemed by the general public as dangerous.

Fact is, whey protein on its own is an awesome nutritional supplement since it is basically powdered milk protein without most of the lactose and fat. Hence, whey protein is an extremely useful source of high-quality protein (a scoop can deliver 10-20 grams), and it is tolerated by those with lactose intolerance and those following a weight-loss diet. Whey protein doesn't contain steroids, illegal stuff or harming substances, and it is a safe supplement that is used by many sedentary people to increase their daily protein intake in a convenient manner.

A scoop in the morning with your milk is an awesome way to start the day, and most whey-protein supplements taste delicious. Like I have advised so enthusiastically throughout this book, do consult your doctor prior to taking a whey protein supplement or making any changes in your nutritional approach.

## 26) What should I do if my hair is at a near-shaved length?

At near-shaved lengths, you can get away with not being as disciplined with your hair grooming and hair care. I'd still advise you to follow the methods and approaches of this book, for the hair that is currently at that near-shaved length will be part of your future great-looking mane were you to grow your hair longer. Moreover, it is best that you get used to optimising the 3 aspects of your hair-management equation as soon as possible.

## 27) I am the mother/father of a boy and would like to manage his hair, should I do anything differently?

First of all, allow me to show you my admiration for having purchased this book with the intent of seeking a follicular solution for your child. It is critical to show one's son at a young age that his hair is part of his self and of who he is. As a boy nears puberty, he starts to realise that his hair is unique to himself, and he may start regarding his hair in a negative manner as at that age boys don't like to be different. Furthermore, most parents prefer to buzz their child's hair because they (parents) don't know how to manage their son's Is, Ss, Es or Zs, which further aggravates the negativity and even hate that a young boy may develop towards his own hair.

You are the pillar of your son's self-embracing. His hair is part of who he is, and the sooner he learns to manage it with your help, the sooner he will understand the stuff atop his head. Remember, humans fear that which they don't understand, so imagine permanently fearing a dead rat at such a young age.

The only difference with regards to his hair-management equation is that you will be providing the management of his 3 aspects for the time being, and I recommend you to slowly get him to do his hair grooming and caring by himself. On top of that, I recommend you to not overload your son with hair products: use a baby shampoo, a mild conditioner and a mild leave-in conditioner. For his styling, use the leave-in conditioner itself or small amounts of a hairstyling agent. Of course, it goes without saying that hair products should only be used at an age in which he is aware of himself and of his hair; if your boy is in his early childhood, only use a baby shampoo to clean his hair and anything else that your paediatric doctor may recommend.

Lastly, since hair type/texture is genetic, be aware that your future children can surprise you with the hair type they inherit. Furthermore, if you have daughters, you can essentially use the same content in this book to manage their hair, though you can certainly take your girls from time to time to a tea house (aka flashy and fabulous hair salon)!

## 28) Can I recommend this book to other people even if they don't look after their hair?

Absolutely. It only takes a male to know how to improve something to become motivated to take charge and improve that something. As you have been able to see for yourself, improving one's hair is not as difficult or elaborate as we males have been brainwashed to believe. In this book, I have made the effort to outline everything in a clear and methodical manner so that all you need is to put the words into action. Any male can benefit from reading this book, and you will be doing a favour to whomever you recommend this book to.

## 29) What should I expect from the opposite sex once I get my hair looking great?

Questions, a lot of questions. Women will flock to you for hair advice; that was the first thing I noticed upon getting my Es optimised. I have had ladies randomly popping out of nowhere in supermarkets, nightclubs and cinemas to ask me a hair question. Initially, the extra female attention is good for stroking your ego and for practising the ancient art of seduction, but it soon grows old as it becomes a daily thing. Of course, always strive to help others regardless of the gender and aim to be part of spreading the word.

In terms of the enhanced attractiveness from achieving your great-looking mane, ever since I started my sites and started spreading the word online, I have continued to get the emails of men all over the world contacting me to thank me. They thank me because they see how their game with the opposite sex (or same sex) improves substantially: women are more open to flirt with them, the bedroom conversion (i.e. going from flirting to the bedroom) is pretty high, and, when they walk into a room or bar, women turn their heads to them.

Women love confidence, full stop. Whether you have Is or Zs for your hair, a bald head or a bushy long mane, women love the self-confidence that a man emanates from having embraced what he has and from having stuck to his principles and beliefs. By finally optimising the stuff atop your head, you are telling people, right there and then, that this is what you have and that you are damn proud of it. This, my friend, is what gets women wet in that special place.

Work on your hair as per this book, and then proceed to work on other aspects of your life. Integrate your great-looking mane into a life full of achievements, and your self-confidence and male status will skyrocket, I guarantee you that.

## 30) I am balding/have started to bald, what do I do?

Two things: embrace it and do something about it.

Embrace your baldness. This means that you should accept that the hair will eventually go. Don't be one of those guys with a combover or with 3 hairs hanging from a ponytail. Deluding yourself will not make you look good in anyone's eyes, not even in your own eyes. Embrace your balding and be positive about yourself; at the end of the day, it is hair, and balding doesn't affect your health, nor does it mean that something is wrong with you. Balding is part of being a male, and about 65% of men are balding profusely by age 60. It will happen to all of us sooner or later if given enough time.

Once you have accepted and embraced your balding, it is then time to do something about it. First of all, start with the hairstyle: no combovers, no long hair, and certainly no hairstyles designed to extravagantly conceal your balding.

If you are a Norwood III or less (i.e. you don't have big balding areas), you can still pretty much sport any of the short and medium-length hairstyles available to non-balding folks although I would encourage you to go for hairstyles that retain length at

209

the front so as to elegantly conceal the receding occurring at the temples. Pay close attention to the term "elegantly"; this means that, when styling your mane, you should allow the hair to smoothly and discreetly hover the receding temples; do not make it look like you are trying too hard. Great hairstyles to elegantly conceal the receding hairline include the Shaggy hairstyle, the Faux Hawk, the Side Fringe, the Jewfro/Afro and the Caesar Cut. All of these hairstyles share the same short to medium-length trait and the emphasis of the hair at the hairline hovering over the receding temples in a discreet and elegant manner.

If you are a Norwood IV or above, go for a short-length trim or buzz, or shave it altogether. At this stage, you will have too much hair-shaft thinning and balding going on at the top, which will only work against your image were you to have your hair longer than a short length. If you don't want to shave your hair because it requires doing it frequently, invest in a hair clipper and go for a #1 up to a #3 all around your head. Cropping your hair like this can be done rapidly and by yourself in the comfort of your own home, so it will be very convenient for you.

Aside from the hair, work on your self-confidence. Lose the emphasis on the hair and instead emphasise other physical attributes of yours. Look neat and polished at all times (including your remaining hair), improve the health of your skin, keep your nails trimmed and clean, brush your teeth frequently, and, last but not least, improve your body. This last one is of special importance because it will not only improve your attractiveness but will also improve your self-confidence and help you to forget about your balding.

Working on your body and getting yourself an awesome body when you are balding is what I call "pulling a Vin Diesel". While Vin Diesel himself is not the best actor around, the man exudes self-confidence and has totally revamped the public's attitude towards balding men for the better. Vin Diesel is a confessed gym addict and looks great, which coupled with his stage persona and self-confidence has garnered him an absurd amount of female followers. Seriously, Vin Diesel appears time and time again on the "hottest males" lists that all those women's magazines love to entertain their readers with, and he shares this privilege with the likes of George Clooney, Matthew McConaughey, Adrian Grenier, Will Smith and Justin Timberlake. Other men who have "pulled a Vin Diesel" include Jason Statham, The Rock and Bruce Willis, so, really, get your awesome body and don't worry about your balding!

Lastly, I have covered the options available to fight against male pattern baldness in the fourth chapter "Hair-Care Aspect: The Big 3 Issues To Battle To Sport Great-Looking Hair", so make sure that you have read these options and understood them. Do remember that currently (as of 2013) there are no options available that will yield permanent and irreversible anti-balding results outside of a hair transplant, and the latter doesn't guarantee said permanent results either. Minoxidil and finasteride only fight MPB for as long as the medications are used; if you stop using them, you will go back to balding, and you will lose any hair that had grown back.

## 31) Is it possible to not use any hair products on my hair?

Yes, it is. I have gone through periods of using no hair products and found this to work for my case. This solo approach is done with the same cleaning, conditioning and styling stages, only that you'd skip the actual shampoo, conditioner and hairstyling agent, solely working the Sebum Coating method for your hair-grooming actions.

If you want to go hair-product solo, you would clean your hair with the mechanical action of your fingers during the Sebum Coating method, you'd condition your hair with your secreted sebum and you would style your mane in your chosen hairstyle without using a hairstyling agent. For what is worth, optimally-spread sebum works as a surprisingly-good hairstyling agent too.

This solo approach to hair grooming works best on short-length hair although you can try this approach at any length. Just take into account that, since you won't be using hairstyling products, most hairstyles won't hold as well or look the same way as they'd do if you used hairstyling agents. Also, be aware that you may require specific shampooing sessions at times when your hair has been exposed to dirt (e.g. you went camping).

The main drawback is that going solo has an important risk of messing it up. If you are are going solo, you will need to master the Sebum Coating method since any excess sebum will not be removed with shampoo, and shampoo is the best hair-cleaning agent to remove important excesses of sebum accumulation. Hence, in order to avoid the potentially-chaotic scenario of having an excessive sebum buildup occurring on your hair, you must master the Sebum Coating method and have your locks sebuminised like you mean business. Likewise, your daily hair-grooming routine may take longer than what it'd otherwise take using hair products, so you have to weigh the pros and cons of going solo.

## 32) Can I use natural or organic hair products too?

Absolutely. You can decide to only use natural oils and butters on your hair, and you can buy your hair products organic if you so prefer. You can also use natural oils and butters while at times using organic products and other times using regular products for your shampooing and conditioning.

Whatever you do, ensure that you abide by the structure of the hair-grooming process and adapt your shampooing frequency and hair-grooming schedule accordingly.

## 33) How can I clean my hair with baking soda and vinegar?

There are 2 common household products that are also useful for cleaning your hair: baking soda and vinegar. These 2 products (used in tandem) act like shampoo and can substitute the shampoo on your shampooing days. Their use, however, is fiddly and requires some experimenting to find out the optimal amounts you'll need as well as their optimal frequency of use. Likewise, the application of these 2 products takes longer than that of shampoo, so you may want to use baking soda and vinegar specifically on some days.

To clean your hair with these 2 kitchen products, first use baking soda. Dilute one tablespoon of the baking soda in one glass of warm water. Then, pour the mix on your hair, aiming to have it poured on your scalp and as per the 6 scalp segments (it will get a bit messy though); once the mix is poured, massage the scalp segments as outlined for the shampooing method. Once you have finished massaging (20-second count per segment), rinse the baking soda thoroughly; failure to rinse it well will result in your hair becoming dry or with white particles. After rinsing the baking soda, pour some vinegar on your scalp and locks (the vinegar being previously diluted), aiming to coat your hair with the vinegar. Once your hair is somewhat soaked in vinegar, then rinse the vinegar with water (from the shower bulb). You may skip the thorough rinsing of the vinegar as the vinegar acts a quasi-conditioner, but the only problem is that your hair may end up giving off a strong vinegar smell; leaving the vinegar on your locks without rising may provide an additional cosmetic benefit to your hair, so experiment with both approaches (i.e. rinsing and not rinsing the vinegar) and gauge the results.

The vinegar must be diluted in a container of warm water, and the optimal amounts to be used for your hair will vary. However, a starting point is to dilute half a cup of vinegar into a litre (or 2 pints) of warm water. Then, you can adjust the dilution gradually as you see it benefits your hair. Furthermore, there's no need to finish the whole 1-litre blend of vinegar and water in one session; you may find that only using half of it works optimally. You can use either white vinegar or apple-cider vinegar, and I recommend you to put each blend (baking soda/water and vinegar/water) in containers that have a lid (e.g. empty shampoo bottles) so that you can pour the blends efficiently.

Pros and cons of using this baking soda/vinegar method as opposed to using shampoo for your hair-cleaning stage?

Pros:

- Works just as good as shampoo under normal conditions (i.e. no heavy excesses of sebum buildup).

- The vinegar surprisingly leaves your hair feeling smooth.

- It is as natural as it gets.

Cons:

- Takes much longer to perform than shampooing alone.

- You still need to do the Sebum Coating method on your non-shampooing days (treat the baking soda/vinegar day as a shampooing day).

- If not rinsed thoroughly, the baking soda may dry your hair or leave white particles behind, and the vinegar may leave your hair smelly (of vinegar).

- Will require adjusting your previously-determined hair-grooming schedule.

- If you're traveling or not at home, this method is difficult to implement.

- Not strong enough to remove accidents with hairstyling agents (e.g. you mistakenly put too much oil on your hair). For bad cases of excessive residue from hairstyling agents or heavy sebum buildup, use shampoo.

This baking soda/vinegar method is to be regarded as a hair-cleaning method and thus as a secondary action to be implemented for your cleaning stage, and it should be considered a shampooing day every time you proceed with this method. However, if you alternate this method with shampooing days (i.e. days where you actually shampoo and use the baking soda/vinegar method on non-shampooing days), then you can skip the conditioning stage and move on to the styling stage any time you perform the baking soda/vinegar method.

All in all, using the baking soda/vinegar method inserts another variable into your hair grooming that will make your hair-grooming routine and schedule more complex. I personally recommend you to stick with the No Shampoo method (i.e. shampoo on shampooing days, Sebum Coating method on non-shampooing days), and then, if you are curious, start playing around with the baking soda/vinegar method, inserting a day here and there.

Whatever you do, always have a structure and follow the hair-grooming process, otherwise you will get lost in the minutiae and end up not achieving the goal of great-looking, convenient hair.

# 34) What are water-soluble hair products and should I use them?

Water-soluble products are products that are supposedly easier to wash off the hair with the Sebum Coating method (i.e. with water and mechanical friction); they are mostly seen with conditioners (both normal and leave-in) as well as quite a few hairstyling agents (most notably pomade and gel). The problem is that, by becoming water soluble, these products tend to have their functionality altered and the hairstyling results they yield tend to be different to those of their conventional counterparts.

Water-based products are most useful if you're going to completely avoid shampoo and will only rely on the Sebum Coating method (or the baking soda/vinegar method) for your long-term hair cleaning. The thing is, with the No Shampoo method integrated into the hair-equation system as you've learnt, you will be self-regulating your hair's cleaning regardless of the hair products you use. For example, if you start using a water-soluble pomade, you will very likely find that your shampooing frequency will be reduced somewhat (i.e. you'll shampoo less frequently) if, prior to the water-soluble pomade, you used to use a conventional pomade. The tradeoff is that water soluble pomades do not adequately provide the "greased" look of conventional pomades, so you will be trading the functionality of regular pomade for a lower shampooing frequency.

What's even equally important to know with water-soluble products is that obtaining good results from them is like playing a roulette. You may find a water-soluble product of more benefit while the dude next to you will abhor that product and will need the conventional form of that product. Likewise, remember that your scalp continues to secrete sebum, so you may find that moving to water-soluble agents doesn't necessarily yield any decrease in shampooing frequency as sebum is what's more important to pay attention to for your hair-grooming efforts.

All of the above is why I tell you to trial different hairstyling agents if you're not happy with your current one and to not to focus on the minutiae that complicates matters even more and is subject to further randomness. Start with a hairstyling product that you like (e.g. one you've used in the past) and grab a shampoo and conditioner as per Question 7. Furthermore, smart application of hairstyling agents and conditioners, which is what you've learnt, is much more important than whether a product is water-soluble or not.

Water-soluble hair products will be advertised as such or as "water based". The water-soluble hair product will have ingredients that are indeed water-soluble and that allow the product to be advertised as such.

## 35) I live in an area with hard water, should I add or do anything else to my hair-care strategy or hair-grooming routine?

If you live in an area with hard water, you may use a chelating shampoo once a month as covered in Chapter 3. However, you may not necessarily need a chelating shampoo as regular shampoos tend to include the chelating agent EDTA anyway. Furthermore, if you have short or medium-length hair and get regular trims, then your need for a chelating shampoo decreases even more.

Hard water can be particularly bad for your kitchen and bathroom, so you could install a water softener in your house and that way not have to worry about hard water affecting your hair or home. If you simply want to avoid hard water at shower time, then you can install a specific shower filter that will catch the dissolved minerals in the hard water.

## 36) I have a skin disorder affecting my scalp, should I follow your book's instructions instead of my dermatologist's instructions?

No. If you have a health/skin disorder affecting your scalp (e.g. scalp psoriasis or seborrheic dermatitis), then you must follow your dermatologist's instructions. Skin disorders affecting the scalp are often treated with medical shampoos, and not using this type of shampoos (or reducing their frequency of use) can deteriorate your scalp. I would, however, encourage you to talk to your dermatologist about the nutritional approach of this book as an optimal intake of omega-3s, zinc and vitamins A and C can potentially help with ameliorating skin disorders.

In the case of dandruff, I still recommend you to visit a dermatologist although you can use an over-the-counter dandruff shampoo to control your dandruff, provided the dandruff is not heavy. Follow the specific instructions of the product and incorporate the indicated frequency of use of the dandruff shampoo to your already worked-out optimal shampooing frequency, inserting the dandruff-shampoo sessions on your "off" days. For example, if you currently have a 1 on/6 off shampooing frequency and your dandruff shampoo calls for its use twice per week, then insert the 2 sessions of dandruff-shampoo use on your "off" days so that, on any 2 of those 6 "off" days of your shampooing frequency, you carry out your dandruff-shampoo sessions. Follow the dandruff shampoo with a normal conditioner unless otherwise stated in the instructions.

## 37) What's the most random hair-related personal story that you have?

When I was living in Dubai (United Arab Emirates), I decided to organise a bodyboarding trip to the seacoast in Oman. Oman is one of the neighbouring countries of the United Arab Emirates, and it has a great coastline in the Arabian Sea with some wicked waves (in bodyboarding, you ride waves lying flat on a board).

I was going with a male friend, and we took my car for what was an approximate 1000-mile drive across part of the Arabian Desert. We decided to stop at a random village for a sleepover as it was getting late and driving at night in Oman is crazy as it is, although the skyline as you drive through the Arabian Desert is absolutely stunning. Once we had checked into the only hotel in the village, my buddy and I decided to visit a nearby shisha bar (Arab smoking bar) that was full of locals in their kandoras (a type of full-body vest) and their keffiyehs (a type of head scarf). As soon as we stepped inside the shisha bar, all the locals turned their heads to look at us.

We shrugged off the attention of the local patrons and went about our business getting a hooka (a smoking device) and some of the funky-smelling tobacco that is smoked with the hooka. I don't smoke, but once in a while hitting a shisha bar is fun, and, despite you don't get high from the stuff, it is a pleasurable experience as you sink into the comfortable seats and chat away with your friends while smoking.

The locals kept staring at us, and one of the things that I have learnt when visiting a new country is to always be extra polite and friendly to the locals if you want them to be on your side. However, the whole staring at us was getting well out of order, and, soon enough, the patrons started to move next to us, forming a circle. Mind you, they actually grabbed their seats and moved themselves close to us without saying a single word and staring at us during the whole process. I looked back at them to know what was going on and found out that all of them were, in fact, looking at me and not at my friend.

217

Homosexuality is banned in Oman, so I knew for sure that we hadn't ended up in a gay bar. The situation was quite worrying because we hardly knew where we were on the map as I had kept driving through a never-ending road that claimed to take us to the Omani seacoast. If something were to happen to us in that shisha bar, nobody would know. The situation was very tense, and I could see through the corner of my eyes how, by now, my buddy stood petrified, and I could swear he had stopped blinking too. We were literally standing in total silence amidst a crowd of about 30 locals who didn't show any facial signs of affection towards us. Moreover, some westerners had been kidnapped recently in Yemen (country next to Oman), so, needless to say, we weren't in the happiest of situations.

Then, I heard a deep masculine voice coming from the back of the bar, asking my friend and I something in Arabic that I didn't understand and that sounded aggressive. Since I hardly spoke Arabic, I then asked politely in English, with my voice trembling but trying to look confident, if he could kindly please repeat what he had said (I emphasised "kindly" and "please" so as to not disturb the angry-sounding local who could potentially kill us and bury our bodies right there). Many westerners have given a bad image of themselves to Omanis, so most locals refuse to speak in English with foreigners and will continue talking in Arabic if they don't like you. I was convinced by now that these guys didn't want to be friends with us.

The aforementioned aggressive-sounding man, somewhere in the invisible back of the bar, then asked me again in Arabic if I spoke Arabic, which I managed to understand, to which I replied (this time in Arabic) that I was sorry but that I didn't speak much of the language. He was addressing me from behind the surrounding crowd, and I could not see him, which added further drama to the situation. He then stepped forward, made his way through the men seating around us and stood in front of me as I remained seated on what, minutes before, was a very comfortable couch.

As soon as he was in front of me, I was able to see how this guy had the bushiest and manliest beard that I had ever seen on anyone, looked about 50 years old and emanated testosterone from every single pore of his skin. Think a darker version of Chuck Norris on a bad day and speaking Arabic.

"I see, my friend", he said, surprising all of us in the room as he had decided to speak those words in English.

218

He paused for a few seconds, the room in total silence. These seconds seemed like an eternity to me, and I just stood there frozen like a bag of broccoli left overnight in the freezer. I was waiting for the bad news despite he had called me his friend.

"You have nice hair, my friend", he then said, breaking the agonising silence that filled the room.

I could not believe it; I was shocked and convinced that he was just giving me a nice compliment to sugarcoat my impending death. He then looked back to the crowd, said something in Arabic, and all the other men started smiling and shouting stuff in joy. The Chuck Norris look-alike then grabbed a chair and sat a mere inches away from me, sporting the biggest and friendliest of smiles.

"What nation you are, my friend?" he asked in broken English.

Still in shock, I managed to say my country of origin. He continued to smile and asked my name; I told him my name, and he then tried to pronounce it, not sounding at all like I had said it (mind you, my name is hard to pronounce as it is). The crowd laughed, and he encouraged me to teach him to pronounce the "-ge" in Rogelio. He got it right on the third attempt.

"You have nice hair, my friend Rogelio."

"Shookran ekteer", I said in Arabic so as to thank him for his kind words.

He smiled as so did the men in the crowd.

He then ordered the guy who was acting as the de facto waiter to bring us more funky tobacco to put on our hookah as well as some huge plates of food for my friend and I to feast on. My new local buddy was literally 2 inches away from me, talking constantly in his broken English while my friend (the one who came with me for the trip) ignored the 2 of us and munched away the food we were brought.

My new buddy was talking about how his sons had hair just like mine and how he would crop their hair to a #2 with a hair clipper that he had. He told me in an amusing manner how his daughters had very curly hair like his and that the girls were always complaining about their hair. While the local traditions frown upon talking about one's wife to another man (especially to a foreigner), he told me that his wife had beautiful straight hair and that he had hoped his daughters would have inherited their mother's hair and not his.

We spent the next 4 hours chatting about hair, hair-related stuff, soccer, local traditions, western culture and joked about our cultural differences. The image that the media in the West gives about Arab people is completely distorted; they made my friend and I feel at home, which is pretty much the same vibe that I have encountered during my life in the Middle East.

We finished off our ramblings and the food devouring, and we went back to our hotel to get some sleep. The next day, we found out that someone had filled up the fuel tank of my car and had cleaned the car's chassis from the desert dust accumulated overnight, all without me knowing anything about it. We also had a box full of water bottles and food waiting for us in the reception of the hotel. As it goes, my new local friend had left a note in reception thanking me for the conversation we had the previous night and for the hair tips and advice I gave him for his children. He had ordered the taking care of my car, the buying for us of provisions for our trip, and he had even sorted out and paid for accommodation for my friend and I to stay in a 4-star hotel in the seaside village we were heading to for our bodyboarding trip! It turned out that he was one of the most respected tribal members in the region, and he had made a few phone calls to make our trip better. Call that luck!

## 38) Are there more things I should know to have a great-looking mane that haven't been covered in all these chapters?

No, not for successfully optimising your hair-management equation. I have written this book with an emphasis on the male who wants a great-looking mane with convenience. You only need to look at the 9-Minute Perfect Mane routine to see the emphasised blend of great results with convenience: you have learnt all the details that go with the actions needed to implement the 9-Minute Perfect Mane routine, and you can easily implement all the actions in 9 minutes or less. I have designed this routine so that you invest 9 minutes of your time to be able to leave your house happy with the stuff atop your head. I could have instead designed a Perfect Mane routine that was attained in 60 minutes, but then, how convenient and relevant would it have been to a modern 21$^{st}$ century male like you and I? What's more is that I have experimented with 60-minute hair-grooming routines and found no real extra benefit from what I could otherwise achieve with a proper 9-minute routine.

I am a strong believer in the Pareto principle. Applied in a non-economic sense, this principle proposes that 80% of results can be achieved with 20% of the 100% of efforts needed to obtain 100% of results. In this book, I bring you exactly this, only that, with this 20% of efforts, you will actually be getting about 95% of results; and that's with 100% of the results being super-duper fabulous diva hair, so you are a mere 5% short of getting your Sex in the City "oh dear, I can't believe it's so luscious" hair. Or, in others words, you are getting your awesome-looking mane (95%), and the remaining 5% is not worth the effort unless you want to remove convenience from your hair-management equation.

Following on from the above, however, I'd like to briefly cover the other things that you can do to tap into the remaining 5% of the aforementioned 100% results.

## Deep condition frequently

Deep conditioning is a form of sealing in extra moisture into the hair and is of special benefit to damaged hair. As you already know, damaged hair occurs from subpar hair care as well as from straightening, relaxing or dying your hair, so you can find some benefit from deep conditioning if you have done any of these 3 actions on your hair and find out that your hair isn't responding as desired to your hair-grooming and hair-care actions.

Because deep conditioning is literally a heavy-duty form of conditioning, it requires more application time and effort than a normal conditioner does, hence it isn't a very convenient hair-conditioning product to use. However, if your current hair has been cared badly or has been straightened, relaxed or dyed, then using a deep conditioner to jump-start your mane-awesomeness journey is advised if you want to keep your current hair; having said that, for best results, I recommend you to instead start your peculiar journey to great-looking, convenient locks with a fresh and virgin batch of hair (i.e. cut your damaged hair).

To use a deep conditioner so as to tap into the remaining 5%, apply the deep conditioner to your hair anywhere from once a week to once a month, and try to do it on your shampooing day, swapping your normal conditioner for the deep conditioner. Likewise, if your current hair (before starting your journey) is/feels dry, you can go by the reactive hair-care measure of deep conditioning your hair every 2 weeks for the next 8 weeks.

## Go into more detail about profiling your hair

I could tell you to also classify your hair according to your strand thickness, protein sensitivity or strand porosity. At the end of the day, however, you'd be even more confused than when you started reading the book and would be feeling like you are reading a manual for girls. Even Anthony himself thinks that doing any more profiling than that covered in the hair-profiling chapter is going way overboard.

All the important stuff that you need to know so as to profile your hair is in this book, and I have written it so that it is especially relevant to the lifestyle-conscious modern male who wants great convenient hair (i.e. you). I have written this book as a modern male for the modern male, and it is my belief that you only need to go as far as the tested basics in hair profiling to further define your hair management and achieve your great-looking mane. I'd rather you put your energy into coming up with your particular hair ID and then move on to master your hair grooming than you waste your stuff with Mickey-Mouse stuff that looks good on paper but has a negligible impact on your hair management as a modern male.

## Split hairs about what goes on when you sleep

I could easily tell you to wear a silk scarf around your head when you go to bed so as to protect your Is, or I could tell you to avoid sleeping on the sides of your head so as to not offset the uber-curvylicious definition of your curls if you have Ss, Es or Zs. By the same token, I could also tell you to sleep vertically and not on a bed because, apparently, this enhances the delta waves produced in the subaquatic region of the phospholipid membrane in the left hemisphere of your brain, and this has been proven to increase concentration levels by 1.1% in sleep-deprived iguanas. At the end of the day, though, you'd have to weigh the pros and cons of what you do.

Sure, when you have your head rubbing against a pillow for 6 to 9 hours, your hair will take some beating. However, I will tell you that impairing your sleep with trivial stuff (e.g. scarves to elaborately protect the hair) will affect your health (including hair) more than any small benefit that obsessing about your mane when you go to bed will yield. Sleep is essential to health and a great life, and optimal sleep should be very high up in your list of priorities, higher than hair actually.

I have done the whole pre-bed routine of covering my mane with weird stuff, soaking my hair in gooish products and more. The result was an uncomfortable night and bad sleep, just to have my curls look a little bit better than if I had gone to bed as I have outlined in this book. You tell me, how am I going to incorporate my optimised hair into a better life if I am failing to get adequate rest and sleep, the latter being one of the foundations to a great life?

As I have suggested in Chapter 4 "Hair-Care Aspect: The Big 3 Issues To Battle To Sport Great-Looking Hair", tie your hair at night into a ponytail or bun if your hair is long enough. If your hair isn't long enough to tie it, you can wear a sleeping cap or do-rag on your head to help minimise the friction on your mane from rubbing your head on the pillow during sleep. If you decide to wear a sleeping cap or do-rag, make sure that it is secured properly and that it doesn't interfere with your sleeping comfort, and you can also coat your locks with some conditioner prior to putting on the sleeping cap or do-rag. Lastly, buy yourself a satin or silk pillow case to minimise head friction, and call it a day. Enjoy your sleep and, when you get up, do the 9-Minute Perfect Mane routine; voila, you have your great-looking mane ready to take the day. Tried, tested and guaranteed.

## Conclusion

Questions will come during your journey; that's for sure. Just about all questions can be answered by referring back to the book, and any miscellaneous questions that crop up will already be answered in this chapter.

You yourself dictate the speed and end of your journey; you're the one who will decide whenever your journey has ended, and you will be basing this decision on how satisfied you are with your hair. You now have all the knowledge you need as well as the plan to succeed in your journey, and no amount of questions will deter you from the right path that you'll be setting once you start putting the knowledge you've learnt into actions.

## Anthony's barbershop case study

Jeremy was a 49-year-old male who had recently divorced. The divorce wasn't smooth, yet the kids seemed to be fine, and they're who matter at the end of the day anyway. Jeremy was going through a second adolescence in that he was now a bachelor again, had an excellent, stable job as a vice-president for a big pharmaceutical company, had all the money in the world, his kids were happy with him and he also had the good looks despite being almost 50. Oh, and he owned a Lamborghini Diablo among other toys of his. In other words, the man was a walking chick magnet, and he was very happy with that.

One of the things Jeremy was working on was in improving his looks, so his hair was one of the things he wanted to optimise. Despite his age, he still had a dense mane of Is, which added to his good looks. He was a regular at Anthony's barbershop, and would come in every week to get a neat trim. However, every time that Jeremy would come in for his weekly visit, he would ask Anthony the same questions on and on. It was quite obvious that Jeremy was getting caught up in the detail and wasn't looking at the big picture.

Anthony and Jeremy had become good friends with all of Jeremy's visit, so Anthony decided to give Jeremy some tough "bro" love and told him to stop asking about Mickey-Mouse stuff and to start concentrating on the essentials of his hair grooming and hair care; essentials that Anthony had repeated numerously in the past but which Jeremy would forget about time and time again. Basically, Anthony wrote up a blunt list of actions for Jeremy to start doing and told him to forget about minutiae for the time being. Anthony told Jeremy to skip the next week's visit and to give himself 2 weeks to concentrate on his hair-grooming essentials before coming back to the barbershop.

Lo and behold, after 2 weeks, Jeremy had made a remarkable improvement with his hair. Jeremy was working on his shampooing frequency and had given himself a week to know his hair in its natural state; his hair already looked better as he had started to optimally coat his hair with his own sebum. Some 6 weeks later, Jeremy's hair was looking so great that, every time he went out on a date with a lady, she would spend part of the date asking him hair questions!

# Epilogue

Well, that's it, my friend; you have reached the end of this book. It is now that you have gone through and garnered all the necessary knowledge to achieve your goal of great-looking, convenient hair. All you have left to do now is to put the same words that you've learnt into actions. Chapter 7 goes through all the steps and actions to take, but a word of caution is needed: ensure to start your journey as soon as you can, for you now have your inner spark flaming (i.e. you are motivated), and this same spark is what will have you waking up every day during your journey to continue implementing actions to get closer to the goal of a great-looking head of Is, Ss, Es or Zs.

Throughout this book, I have emphasised convenience; you have seen this convenience in the form of the 9-Minute Perfect Mane routine, which has you every day getting your hair looking as you want it to look in mere minutes. In fact, convenience is just as crucial as obtaining the great looks of your hair because hair grooming must be done every day, which means that there is no way you'd be able to otherwise groom your hair with an inconvenient routine or hair-management system. The 9-Minute Perfect Mane routine is just another essential piece of your hair-management equation and one that is integrated with the rest of your hair-grooming elements and hair-management aspects.

Your journey to mane awesomeness is one that will be pleasurable; you will enjoy every action that you implement for you will be able to see instant results, which will then continue to keep you motivated to reach your goal of finally being happy with your great-looking hair. Don't worry about how long it takes; worry about improving your hair gradually and seeing frequent results from the hair-management actions you implement every day. As mentioned in the seventh chapter, it can take you between 5 weeks to 17 weeks to have your hair perfectly customised to your desire and to have you finally happy with your mane. The good thing is that, once you have achieved your goal, that same great-looking hair will stay atop your head for the many years ahead and your hair-management efforts will be on auto-pilot.

I trust that you will achieve your goal; the same way that I have trusted others who, with my help, have also achieved their great-looking manes and have finally been happy with their hair. I know the effort that it takes to achieve great-looking hair, which is why the system that you have learnt has you constantly implementing actions that yield positive results so as to reinforce your desire and motivation. All in all, you have everything in your power to succeed and add another achievement to your life.

Without you, this book would be just another book. I encourage you to spread the word and to act to inspire and motivate others into doing something positive about their hair. You are now in a position to pass on the word and help others achieve their great-looking, convenient manes too. The vast majority of men are walking around with dead rats and buzz cuts, not because they want to but because they don't know how to do otherwise. It is time we altogether break the silly notions that surround male hair and help each other to become better.

For now, our meeting points are my sites Manly Curls and Men's Hair Blog, and you can find me on Twitter and Facebook too.

http://www.manlycurls.com/          http://www.menshairblog.com/

http://www.facebook.com/ManlyCurls          https://twitter.com/ManlyCurls

You can keep in touch with me, and I invite you to keep me updated on your progress.

Just like I did with my previous book, I have left this last paragraph that you are now reading till the end of the book's writing. These are now my last word, and I want to use them to first say that I have thoroughly enjoyed writing this book. It is my second book, so I'm very happy to have completed another literary hair-related resource and now be able to share it with you. Most of all, I want to thank you for having purchased my book and for believing in my message. Just like you believe in my message, I believe in you, and I'm sure that you will be joining the ranks of us men who are finally happy with the stuff atop their heads.

Stay strong and determined, my friend.

All the best.

Rogelio

# APPENDIX

## Appendix I – The hair-management equation

| HAIR-MANAGEMENT EQUATION | | |
|---|---|---|
| *Hair profiling* | *Hair Grooming* | *Hair care* |
| Hair basics | Cleaning | Dry hair |
| Hair type | Conditioning | Tangled hair |
| Hair lengths | Styling | Hair loss |
| Curl Factor | Hair grooming routine | Proactive/Reactive measures |
| Norwood stage | Hair products | Nutrition |

| HAIR PROFILING | | | |
|---|---|---|---|
| Hair type | Hair lengths | Curl Factor | Norwood stage |

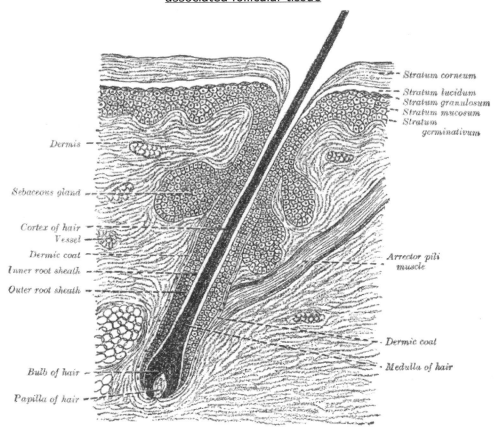

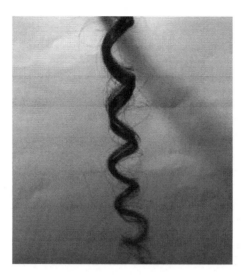

| TEXTURES | |
| --- | --- |
| *Non-Curly* | *Curly* |
| Straight hair | Wavy hair |
| | Coiled hair |
| | Kinky hair |

FRONT OF HEAD

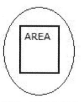

BACK OF HEAD

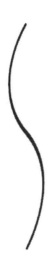

$\mathcal{E}$

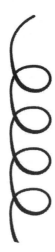

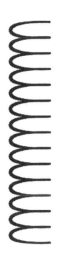

| | HAIR TYPES | | | |
|---|---|---|---|---|
| | STRAIGHT | WAVY | COILED | KINKY |
| Hair shape | Straight linear shape | Wave-like shape | Coiled and spiral-like shape | Coiled and tightly-angled shape |
| Alphabetical resemblance | I | S | E | Z |

| HAIR LENGTHS ELEMENT | | |
|---|---|---|
| Extended hair length | Visible hair length | Extended length category |

| EXTENDED HAIR LENGTH | |
|---|---|
| *Hair length (inches)* | *Hair length category* |
| Less than 0.125 | Near-shaved |
| 0.125 – 2 | Short |
| 2 – 6 | Medium |
| Over 6 | Long |

| Hair type | Curl Factor |
|---|---|
| Straight hair | 1-1.1 |
| Wavy hair | 1.11-1.5 |
| Coiled hair | 1.51-2.5 |
| Kinky hair | 2.51+ |

## Appendix XVI – Damp vs. Dry effect according to hair type and extended hair length (general guideline)

| Hair length | HAIR TYPES | | | |
|---|---|---|---|---|
| | *Straight* | *Wavy* | *Coiled* | *Kinky* |
| Short | Barely | Barely | Mild | Moderate |
| Medium | Barely | Mild | Moderate | Intense |
| Long | Barely | Mild | Moderate | Intense |

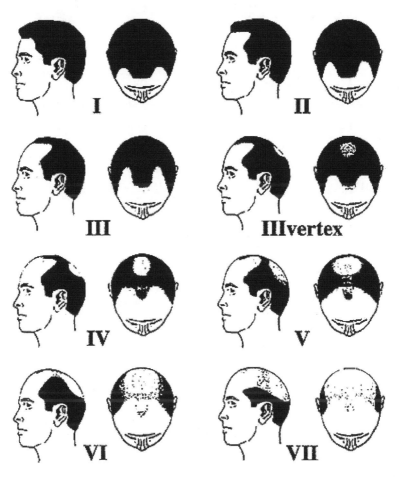

*Image credit: Dr. O'Tar Norwood, Southern Medical Journal, Issue 11, Vo. 68, 1975*

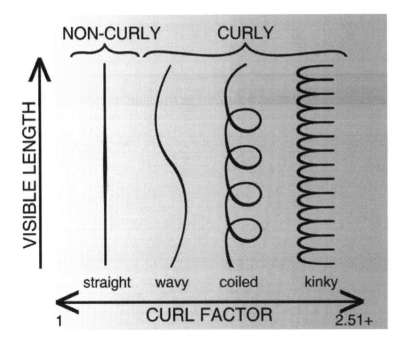

| STAGES | SECONDARY ACTIONS | | | |
|---|---|---|---|---|
| Cleaning | Use Shampoo | Sebum Coating method | | |
| Conditioning | Use normal conditioner | Sebum Coating method | Skip conditioning | |
| Styling | Use leave-in conditioner | Use hairstyling agent/s | Put hair into hairstyle | Dry hair |

247

<u>Appendix XX – Typical shampooing frequency per hair type and extended length</u>
<u>category (High= 1 on/1 off, Very low= 1 on/7 off)</u>

| | HAIR TYPES | | | |
|---|---|---|---|---|
| | *Straight* | *Wavy* | *Coiled* | *Kinky* |
| Near-shaved | High | High | Medium | Medium |
| Short | High | Moderate | Moderate | Low |
| Medium | High | Moderate | Low | Low |
| Long | Moderate | Low | Low | Very low |

| STAGES | SHAMPOOING DAY | NON-SHAMPOOING DAY |
|---|---|---|
| *Cleaning* | Shampoo | Sebum Coating method (dual action) |
| *Conditioning* | Normal conditioner | |
| *Styling* | Yes | Yes |
| *Leave-in conditioner?* | No (style with other hairstyling agent) | Yes (style with leave-in + other hairstyling agent) |

<u>Appendix XXII – A straight line (i.e. non-curly hair) and a non-straight line (i.e. curly hair)</u>

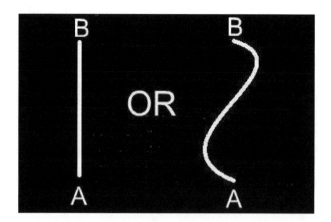

# Appendix XXIII – Timespan in months growing from a shaved length (0 inches) to stipulated visible lengths

|  | Shaved | 2 inches | 4 inches | 6 inches | 12 inches |
|---|---|---|---|---|---|
| Straight | 0 | 4 | 8 | 12 | 24 |
| Wavy | 0 | 6 | 12 | 18 | 36 |
| Coiled | 0 | 10 | 20 | 30 | 60 |
| Kinky | 0 | 12 | 24 | 36 | 72 |

|  | Shaved | 2 inches | 4 inches | 6 inches | 12 inches |
|---|---|---|---|---|---|
| Straight | 0 | 2 | 4 | 6 | 12 |
| Wavy | 0 | 3 | 6 | 9 | 18 |
| Coiled | 0 | 5 | 10 | 15 | 30 |
| Kinky | 0 | 6 | 12 | 18 | 36 |

# Appendix XXV – Example of a weekly schedule according to a 1 on/1 off shampooing frequency

| | Monday | Tuesday | Wednesday | Thursday | Friday | Saturday | Sunday |
|---|---|---|---|---|---|---|---|
| Shampoo | On | Off | On | Off | On | Off | On |
| Sebum Coating method | Off | On | Off | On | Off | On | Off |
| Conditioner | On | Off | On | Off | On | Off | On |
| Leave-in (as styling agent) | Off | On | Off | On | Off | On | Off |
| Style | Yes | Yes | Yes | Yes | Yes | Yes | Yes |
| Time Taken (minutes) | 8.7 mins | 4.5 mins | 8.7 mins | 4.5 mins | 8.7 mins | 4.5 mins | 8.7 mins |

| | HAIR TYPES | | | |
|---|---|---|---|---|
| | *STRAIGHT* | *WAVY* | *COILED* | *KINKY* |
| Hair shape | Straight linear shape | Wave-like shape | Coiled and spiral-like shape | Coiled and tightly-angled shape |
| Curls? | No. Occasional bending at 3+ inches | Yes. Forms loose curls (i.e. waves) | Yes. Forms tight curls that express as coils | Yes. Extremely-tight curls not discernible from distance |
| Alternative technical name | Non-curly | Curly | Curly | Curly |
| Alphabetical resemblance | I | S | E | Z |
| Curl Factor range (typical) | 1 – 1.1 | 1.11 – 1.5 | 1.51 – 2.5 | 2.51+ |
| Male References | Brad Pitt/Tom Cruise/Justin Bieber | George Clooney/Antonio Banderas/Adrian Grenier | Justin Timberlake/ Kenny G/Corbin Bleu | Lenny Kravitz/Will Smith/Kofi Annan |
| Shampooing frequency | High | Medium | Low | Low |
| Need for extra conditioning | Low | Medium | High | High |

| | SHORT-LENGTH HAIR (UP TO 2 INCHES) | | | |
| --- | --- | --- | --- | --- |
| | Straight | Wavy | Coiled | Kinky |
| Shampoo | 1 on 1 off | 1 on 1 off | 1 on 2 off | 1 on 3 off |
| Conditioner | Every shampooing day | Every shampooing day | Every shampooing day + 50% off days | Every shampooing day + 50% off days |
| Sebum Coating method | Every non-shampooing day | Every non-shampooing day | Every non-shampooing day | Every non-shampooing day |
| Leave-in | Every non-shampooing day | Every non-shampooing day | Every non-shampooing day | Every non-shampooing day |
| Hairstyling agents | Wax/Pomade /Gel/Mousse | Wax/Pomade /Gel/Mousse | Leave-in/Gel/Oils/Styling creams/Pomade | Leave-in/Oils/Styling cream |
| Combing | Conventional comb/Wide-tooth comb/Fingers | Wide-tooth comb/Fingers | Wide-tooth comb/Fingers | Wide-tooth comb/Fingers |
| Suitable hairstyle | Spikes | Caesar Cut | Faux Hawk | High and Tight |
| Tangling risk | Low | Low | Low | Moderate |
| Ability to puff out | Low | Low | Moderate | High |
| Damp vs. Dry Effect | Barely | Barely | Mild | Moderate |
| Drying method | Towel/Finger Shakeout | Towel/Finger Shakeout | Towel/Finger Shakeout | Towel/Finger Shakeout |

| | MEDIUM-LENGTH HAIR (UP TO 2 INCHES) | | | |
| --- | --- | --- | --- | --- |
| | Straight | Wavy | Coiled | Kinky |
| Shampoo | 1 on 1 off | 1 on 2 off | 1 on 3 off | 1 on 4 off |
| Conditioner | Every shampooing day | Every shampooing day | Every shampooing day + 50% off days | Every shampooing day + 75% off days |
| Sebum Coating method | Every non-shampooing day | Every non-shampooing day | Every non-shampooing day | Every non-shampooing day |
| Leave-in | Every non-shampooing day | Every non-shampooing day | Daily | Daily |
| Hairstyling agents | Wax/Pomade /Gel/Mousse/ Spray | Wax/Pomade /Gel/Mousse/ Leave-in | Leave-in/Gel/Oils/Styling cream/Pomade | Leave-in/Oils/Styling cream/Pomade |
| Combing | Conventional comb/Wide-tooth comb/Fingers | Wide-tooth comb/Fingers | Wide-tooth comb/Fingers | Wide-tooth comb/Fingers |
| Suitable hairstyle | Shaggy | Side Swept | Jewfro | Afro |
| Tangling risk | Low | Moderate | Moderate | High |
| Ability to puff out | Low | Moderate | Moderate | High |
| Damp vs. Dry Effect | Barely | Mild | Moderate | Intense |
| Drying method | Towel/Shake out | Towel/Finger Shakeout | Towel/Finger Shakeout | Towel/Finger Shakeout |

256

| | LONG-LENGTH HAIR (OVER 6 INCHES) | | | |
|---|---|---|---|---|
| | *Straight* | *Wavy* | *Coiled* | *Kinky* |
| *Shampoo* | 1 on 2 off | 1 on 3 off | 1 on 5 off | 1 on 6 off |
| *Conditioner* | Every shampooing day | Every shampooing day + 50% off days | Every shampooing day + 75% off days | Every shampooing day + 75% off days |
| *Sebum Coating method* | Every non-shampooing day | Every non-shampooing day | Every non-shampooing day | Every non-shampooing day |
| *Leave-in* | Daily | Daily | Daily | Daily |
| *Hairstyling agents* | Pomade/Gel/ Mousse/Spray/Leave-in | Pomade/Gel/ Mousse/Leave-in/Spray | Leave-in/Gel/Oils/Styling cream/Pomade | Leave-in/Oils/Styling cream |
| *Combing* | Conventional comb/Wide-tooth comb/Fingers | Wide-tooth comb/Fingers | Wide-tooth comb/Fingers | Wide-tooth comb/Fingers |
| *Suitable hairstyle* | Shoulder Length | Jim Morrison | Beyond Shoulder Length | Braids |
| *Tangling risk* | Moderate | Moderate | High | High |
| *Ability to puff out* | Low | Low | Moderate | High |
| *Damp vs. Dry Effect* | Barely | Mild | Moderate | Intense |
| *Drying method* | Towel/Shake out | Towel/Finger Shakeout | Towel/Finger Shakeout | Towel/Finger Shakeout |

Made in the USA
Lexington, KY
15 September 2018